The ALLERGY-FREE Baby & Toddler Book

The definitive guide to understanding and managing your child's food allergy

CHARLOTTE MUQUIT & DR ADAM FOX

Vermilion
LONDON

1 3 5 7 9 10 8 6 4 2

First published in 2014 by Vermilion, an imprint of Ebury Publishing
A Random House Group company

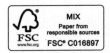

Printed and bound in Great Britain by Clays Ltd, St Ives PLC

ISBN 9780091954871

To buy books by your favourite authors and register for offers visit
www.randomhouse.co.uk

The information in this book has been compiled by way of general guidance in relation to
the specific subjects addressed, but is not a substitute and not to be relied on for medical,
healthcare, pharmaceutical or other professional advice on specific circumstances and in
specific locations. So far as the author is aware the information given is correct and up to
date as at April 2014. Practice, laws and regulations all change, and the reader should ob-
tain up to date professional advice on any such issues. The author and publishers disclaim,
as far as the law allows, any liability arising directly or indirectly from the use, or misuse,
of the information contained in this book.

Contents

Acknowledgements

Many people have helped in the creation of the book.

Adam would like to thank all of the patients that he sees in his allergy clinic, for being a continued source of both education and inspiration.

Many families have helped by sharing their stories. All of the children in this book have, or are suspected of having, a food allergy – some have a diagnosis and some are in the earlier stages of discovery. Each family has a story to tell and each unique journey has a lesson for you, the reader, regardless of where you are on that journey. Every story points towards the importance of inclusion, consideration and understanding in order to make life easier for the child who is living with an allergy. Let me introduce the families:

- Emma is the mum of twins, Cameron and Dillon, aged four.
- Emma Kelly is the mum of Hunter, aged two.
- Thanh is the mum of Charlie, aged 18 months.
- Hannah is the mum of a little boy who she does not want to name. He is aged 16 months. We will call him S.
- Bev is the mum of Levi, aged four.
- Emily is the mum of Felix, aged one, Finn, aged four and Leo, aged eight.
- Erica is the mum of Evan, aged seven.
- Mel is the mum of a little girl, E, aged seven.
- Anne is the mum of Hannah and Edward, aged almost five and two.

- Kathryn is the mum of Sam, aged four and Harry, aged one.
- Sam is the mum of Alex, aged four.
- Brandy is the mum of Kobe, aged three.

The experiences of these families are shared throughout this book. While reading their stories, I was touched by each experience and the joys and agonies that they bring. Their input and insights have brought this book to life. It was also a pleasure and privilege to meet many of the children. So a huge thank you is due to all of those who revisited early painful memories and offered their time, thoughts and recipes in order for this book to be completed.

I would also like to thank:

Sam Muquit for making me laugh, proofreading and for trying my food. Dr and Mrs Haworth for their support, editing and time.

My lovely friends including Jules Ellis, Heidi Messias, Jo Hastings, Rachel Tomasevic, Anna Walsh and Rochelle Rouse, who have encouraged and supported me and helped make everyday life and socialising with Zach an easy and good experience.

Dr Adam Fox, consultant paediatric allergist, who provided endless support and encouragement.

Thanh Thai for the initial 'blue sky thinking'!

Rachel De Boer, paediatric allergy dietician, for her knowledge, advice, encouragement and time.

Philippa Sitters, Jane Graham Maw and Jennifer Christie at Graham Maw Christie Literary Agents.

Catherine Knight and Susanna Abbott at Random House.

Who Are We and Why Did We Write This Book?

My name is Charlotte and I am the mum of a little boy who has multiple food allergies, hay fever and asthma. My decision to write this book came partly through my personal need to write down my experiences of my allergic little boy, aimed at no one in particular, and partly through a desire that no one should go through my family's suffering and, most importantly, my little boy's suffering, because of undiagnosed food allergies. The amount of pain, tears and heartache my husband and I went through watching our baby suffer, and the ignorance and lack of information we experienced when help and support should have been readily available, was almost unbearable.

Food allergies in children are not uncommon. They are, in fact, on the increase. Once diagnosed, management is straightforward and the child's quality of life improves dramatically. Life with a child with food allergies has its challenges but it is not horrendous, nor hopeless. With timely support and accurate advice I believe that my little boy's start in life would have been peaceful and calm. I also would have had more of a chance to enjoy becoming the mum that I always wanted to be.

My hope is that this book becomes a source of support, help and much more to you. It contains information, practical advice, recipes and tips to help smooth the journey from diagnosis to management of food allergies. This book is also an invaluable resource for grandparents, friends and childcare providers as it offers emotional and practical advice to help support the child and their family. The stories of the families that you will find in this book are invaluable, unique and personal. The journey through food allergies does not have to be a lonely one. There is a whole community of families out there, each with different stories, all hoping to achieve the same thing – a balanced, involved, happy and safe life for their child.

Dr Adam Fox is a consultant paediatric allergist and clinical lead for Allergy at Guy's and St Thomas' Hospital and a medical advisor to both Allergy UK and the Anaphylaxis Campaign. He was recently named among Britain's top 250 doctors (*Tatler*, January 2013) and included in 'The Times Magazine: Britain's Best Children's Doctors' (2012). He was awarded 'Paediatric Allergist of the Year' by Allergy UK in 2007.

His clinical role involves the management of children with multiple allergic disease, including food allergy, asthma and rhinoconjunctivitis, as well as children with difficult eczema where food allergy plays a role.

I first contacted Adam when I saw his name in a baby-weaning book. I sent him an email with my book proposal out of the blue and he was supportive and enthusiastic about it from the start. We then met in person when my husband and I took Zach to see him in his London clinic. We had been struggling with our local allergy service for months and felt that we were no clearer and making no progress with Zach's allergies. Zach was nearly two years old by then and we had been managing his allergies with our local services since he was eight months. However, unfortunately it felt like we had been left to it. Despite six-monthly reviews, there was no plan and very limited support. Adam was brilliant, ordering repeat blood tests and doing skin prick tests there and then. He provided medical safety information for when Zach started at preschool and, most importantly, gave us pointers as to where Zach may be heading in terms of allergies and at what age he may grow out of them. More than anything, I had always thought that allergy management could be quite straightforward, with regular reviews, occasional tests and otherwise food avoidance, yet we had never actually experienced anything other than confusion and guesswork from our local service. Adam provided something concrete when we saw him and a definite structure to follow, which gave us a great sense of reassurance and allowed us to get on with our roles as parents.

It is important to point out that this book is not a medical book, nor does it aim to replace the role of the healthcare professional. The early involvement of your GP and referral to an allergy specialist and dietician to oversee the diagnosis and management of your child's food allergies is essential. Nothing can replace the expertise of the people who have trained and who work within the medical field and more specifically the specialty of childhood allergy. This book is, however, a guide to help you through the first few years, to point you towards the healthcare professionals and provide useful advice and support from parents in a similar situation. It is written through personal experience by a mum with the support of an allergy expert. The quotes used in this book represent the real-life experiences of the parents that we spoke to who readily shared their stories. They are intended to illustrate and share what other families have been through, but might not mirror your own experiences exactly. They also do not necessarily represent the views of the authors. To make the most of this book, read a section as it becomes relevant to you and your child. Our website, which accompanies this book, contains helpful images and illustrations of allergic symptoms, reactions and the recipes. You will find it at www.allergyfreebabyandtoddler.com. The hope is that this book will act as a quick-reference guide for you to help promote the safe and efficient management of your child's food allergies and so improve your own and your child's overall quality of life.

Introduction

The past few decades have seen a huge rise in allergic diseases, particularly in the Western world, with recent studies suggesting that almost half of British children have some form of allergic problem, such as asthma, eczema or hay fever during their lives. Allergic disease is the umbrella term that covers food allergy, eczema, asthma and allergic rhinitis. This book was originally written about food allergy because, when Zach was diagnosed with food allergy, I found that there was very little good information and support available. I soon discovered that, although I had never experienced food allergy among my friends or family, Zach was not alone and that more and more children are being affected. Once considered to be something of a rare curiosity, food allergy now affects over 5 per cent of children in the UK. The number of children put on restricted diets by their parents because of a presumed allergy is thought to be much higher. This book now covers numerous other aspects of allergic disease, not just food allergy. Eczema, asthma and allergic rhinitis are also discussed, as their appearance and management are often part and parcel of the life and experience of a child with food allergy.

Most serious food allergies start in infancy and early childhood. They are caused by a relatively small number of foods and often tend to disappear during the course of childhood.

It is important to know that any child who is believed to have a food allergy would benefit from being seen at a specialist children's allergy clinic, where a medical history can be taken, and an examination and allergy testing performed. This allows a formal diagnosis to be made.

Your child's story is the cornerstone of accurate diagnosis of a food allergy and will guide the clinician as to what allergy tests are needed.

Being diagnosed with a food allergy has a massive impact on the whole family. Eating is such a central part of daily life that having to be absolutely sure a child has no contact with a particular food must inevitably affect mealtimes, school, holidays and social occasions. As the parent, you need to be able to recognise reactions and know exactly how to deal with them when they occur. This usually involves carrying antihistamines and possibly adrenaline injectors everywhere the child goes. Children with food allergies can also be at risk of missing out on essential nutrients if they are not properly advised.

Unfortunately, there appears to be no cure for food allergies on the immediate horizon, although promising research, such as work on food desensitisation, does promise real progress over the next few years, not only in the understanding of how to prevent allergies in the first place, but in helping those who already have them.

If there is no cure as yet, there is still plenty that can be done. Through the use of other families' experiences, we hope that this book will be a great resource for not only the parents and carers of children with food allergies, but also any childcare provider and for healthcare professionals who work with such children. Allergies are diverse in how they show themselves, in how your child will react and how distressed and ill they will be. While you find out more about your child's allergies, we hope that this book will provide sensible advice to guide you through the process with pointers to look out for, information to seek from medical professionals, tips on how to cope, support for when you cannot cope and recipes to take away the added stress of an impending birthday or Christmas celebration. All of this, it is hoped, will improve your quality of life, decrease your stress and tiredness levels and allow the first few years of life to be the wonderful experience that they should be.

CHAPTER 1
What is a Food Allergy?

So what exactly is a food allergy and how is that different to a food intolerance, for example? The definitions and terms used can be confusing. Being informed and understanding some 'allergy speak' before you attend healthcare appointments can help in the process of diagnosing and managing your child's allergies. In order to understand how allergies are diagnosed, it is essential to be clear about what is meant by food allergy and food intolerance. It is also important to know how your child may look and behave when reacting to a food, how to go about getting a diagnosis and how to manage the symptoms.

Although many people (and healthcare professionals) may use terms such as allergy and intolerance interchangeably, they do have strict medical definitions. However, despite these definitions, the terminology causes much confusion and many things that are neither an allergy nor an intolerance are still labelled as such. With children, colic, colds, teething, wind, sleep disturbance, runny or strange-coloured nappy contents and infections are all quite common and may be caused by problems with food, but more commonly are not. As a parent, the process of working out what is common and what is not can be very difficult.

This chapter will try to start to smooth the process of diagnosing your child with a food allergy. The hope is to empower you to be able to talk knowledgeably to the healthcare professionals, and to know the direction in which you are heading, in terms of diagnosis and management.

It is essential to get professional help if you suspect that your child may have a food allergy as even though there is no cure, food allergies can be managed. But first you need a diagnosis so that the suspect food can be removed from your child's diet. It is, however, not as easy as it sounds. Great care must be taken when removing any food from your child's diet, as improper diagnosis could lead to an unnecessarily restricted diet and, in the extreme, cause malnutrition. While it is terrible for your child to eat the wrong foods, it is also unhelpful to needlessly deny the right foods. If your child's diet is to be restricted anyway, it is no help to restrict it further than it needs to be. Correct diagnosis is key in the case of suspected allergy.

Chapters 2 and 3 will lead you to take the correct steps towards the diagnosis of a food allergy, but first let's start with some definitions.

Definitions

Allergy: An inappropriate, overreaction of the immune system to a harmless substance (referred to as an allergen) such as dust mite, animal hair, pollen or food.

Food allergy: An inappropriate immune response to a particular food protein. Food allergy can be either IgE mediated (immediate type) or non-IgE mediated (delayed type).

IgE mediated food allergy: These are known as immediate type allergies because they happen very quickly after the food is eaten. Reactions are caused by the immune system causing the body to release histamine and other chemicals, leading to hives, swelling and, in rare cases, anaphylaxis (a severe, life-threatening reaction). Skin prick or blood-specific IgE testing are useful for making a diagnosis. See Chapter 2 for more on this type of allergy.

Non-IgE mediated food allergy: These are known as delayed type allergies because the reaction does not occur until some hours (or even days) after the food is eaten, making them very difficult to diagnose. The reaction is caused by a different part of the immune system to IgE mediated reactions and does not involve allergic antibodies or histamine release. As a result the symptoms are quite different and are often the result of the child continuing to eat the food that they are allergic to. Delayed allergies are mainly a problem in young children and outgrown by early childhood, with cow's milk being the most common cause. One of the biggest problems is diagnosis as allergy tests are unhelpful for delayed allergy. See Chapter 3 for more on this type of allergy.

Anaphylaxis or anaphylactic reaction: Rapid onset of severe symptoms involving more than one organ system that can occur with IgE mediated food allergy. Rare but potentially life-threatening, anaphylaxis or anaphylactic reaction is a medical emergency. See Chapter 8 for more on this type of allergy.

Food intolerance: More common than a food allergy, food intolerance is a reaction to food that does not involve the immune system. Although the symptoms of intolerance can mimic those of allergy, the causes are different and the onset of symptoms is often slower and longer lasting.

Atopic disease: A group of illnesses, including eczema, hay fever, food allergy and asthma that are characterised by the presence of immunoglobulin E (IgE) antibodies.

Terms such as food allergy, food intolerance and food hypersensitivity are often used interchangeably, even though they are very different conditions. To try to clear the confusion, modern classifications have divided reactions to food into those that are immune mediated such as food allergy and those that are not immune mediated, such as food intolerance.

Despite clear classification systems, the term food intolerance is still incorrectly used and understood by healthcare professionals and the general public for the group of delayed allergic reactions to food that are non-IgE mediated. The common use of the term 'cow's milk intolerance', often used to describe non-IgE mediated immunological reactions to cow's milk, illustrates this point well. Referring to a delayed allergic reaction to cow's milk protein as an intolerance allows for further blurring and confusion with lactose intolerance – an entirely different issue.

Intolerance to lactose in cow's milk, is a non-immunological condition present in most of the world's adult population but less so in Caucasians. The age of onset, previous history of milk tolerance and symptoms of bloating and diarrhoea, linked to the amount of milk consumed, make it relatively easy to distinguish from a true allergy to cow's milk.

Food Intolerance
• •

Symptoms of food intolerance can include almost anything but most commonly fatigue and gastrointestinal symptoms, such as diarrhoea and vomiting, bloating (often as part of irritable bowel syndrome) are described.

Causes

The causes of food intolerance can be a chemical substance in the food that your child's body reacts to, a toxic substance produced by some foods that your child reacts to, a food additive, or alternatively, your child can lack the enzymes that are needed to break some foods down.

For young children, lactose intolerance can be a short-lived problem that occurs following a stomach virus. A stomach virus may temporarily damage the gut lining where the lactase enzyme is usually stored. Once recovered, the lining is able to digest the lactose again. This is why your GP may advise you to avoid milk and milk products for your child for a number of days after this type of illness. However, lactose intolerance can also be present from birth with no apparent cause and this variety makes it difficult to identify although this is extremely rare. This book does not cover food intolerance, only allergy. If you suspect that your child has a food intolerance, please liaise with your GP. Most of the time a GP can diagnose food intolerance from a detailed history and refer your child to a dietician if necessary.

Food intolerance or delayed allergy?

Unfortunately, food intolerance can often be confused with delayed food allergy because the symptoms are similar. It is very difficult to identify the cause of a delayed food allergy as symptoms can present hours or days after ingestion. Food diaries (see page 262) are helpful in the diagnosis but only in trying to identify an improvement in symptoms when the suspect allergen is removed and again when it is reintroduced. Allergy tests are typically negative and without the input of an experienced physician it can take an inordinately long time for a diagnosis to be made.

> *When I think about our family's journey into diagnosing Charlie's cow's milk [delayed] allergy I cannot believe how long it actually took and how unhelpful the first-line medical professionals actually were.*
>
> THANH, MUM OF CHARLIE

Oral Allergy Syndrome

Oral Allergy Syndrome usually occurs later in childhood or into adulthood. It happens after a person develops an allergy to pollen (such as grass or tree pollen allergy – otherwise known as hay fever). As well as getting seasonal symptoms, the immune system may start recognising foods containing proteins that have a very similar structure to the pollen. When the food is consumed, the immune system mistakenly sees it as being pollen and causes a mild allergic reaction in the mouth. This can happen with food that has previously been regularly eaten without any problem at all. So, for example, an allergy to the pollen from a birch tree may result in an allergy to eating apple, peach, plum, cherry, potato, carrot, hazelnut, pumpkin seed and aubergine. There is also ragweed pollen allergy, which can cause a reaction to melon and banana, mugwort (celery, tomato) and grass-pollen allergies (tomato, melon and peach).

These reactions are very rarely severe and usually limited to itching around the mouth with mild swelling. The process of digestion or cooking the food quickly destroys these pollen-like proteins, so generally a person has a mild response or no response to the cooked food. For example, a child with oral allergy symptoms to apple will be able to consume apple pie or processed apple juice. Other factors such as the ripeness of the fruit, peeling it or even the presence of hay fever symptoms can all influence the reactions. However, while some reactions to nuts, such as hazelnuts or peanuts, can be due to this pollen cross-reactivity, they may also be due to potentially serious reactions so always discuss what has occurred with your doctor. Simple testing can helpfully differentiate the potentially serious from the irritating but much less dangerous reactions.

The Immune System

Food allergy is an inappropriate immune response to a harmless substance in food. Our immune system is designed to protect the body from harm and disease through identifying harmful or foreign substances that we eat, drink or inhale and then destroying them. Knowing how the immune system works will help you to understand the allergy tests and what the healthcare professionals are looking for when diagnosing your child.

The immune system is designed to protect the body from harmful bacteria, viruses and parasites. One way that it does this is by making proteins called immunoglobulins (Ig). The immunoglobulin often involved in food allergy is called IgE. Children who inherit allergic genes from their parents (although sometimes they seem to appear from nowhere) have an immune system that tends to produce IgE in response to different proteins that should, in fact, be ignored. This tends to happen with the same proteins in most children who have an allergic or 'atopic' tendency to foods such as milk, egg and nuts or to pollen, dust mites or animal hair. Often, the production of IgE doesn't turn into a real allergy, although the IgE can still be seen on an allergy test. We don't understand what makes the difference between children who produce IgE to milk yet are fine when they drink it and those who have an allergic reaction – sometimes the only way to tell them apart is to see what happens when they are exposed.

Most serious food allergies start in infancy and early childhood. They are caused by a relatively small number of different foods (see Chapter 2) and tend to disappear by themselves during childhood. Other common food allergens vary depending on where you live. While peanut and tree nut allergies are common in the US, UK and Australia, fish and seafood allergies are more common in South-East Asia and Southern Europe. Other common problem foods include wheat, soy, sesame seeds and kiwi fruit.

What happens to the body during an allergic reaction?

During a food allergic reaction, the food is eaten and protein in that food is recognised by the IgE that the immune system has previously (and inappropriately) produced. The IgE then triggers what healthcare professionals call an IgE mediated immune response, an allergic reaction. The IgE activates other cells in lots of different places around the body. These other cells contain histamine and other similar chemicals and are responsible for the visible signs that you see on your child during a reaction. Cells releasing histamine in the skin cause hives and swelling; those in the breathing system cause tightening of the airways in the neck and lungs (much like asthma); and those in the stomach and bowel cause vomiting and diarrhoea. Unfortunately, while most reactions are mild and limited to the site of contact (the mouth), sometimes the reaction causes a cascade, where the activation of some cells begins the activation of others. The danger is that a huge response is triggered, resulting in a severe allergic reaction – anaphylaxis (see Chapter 8).

As we mentioned earlier, not all reactions are IgE mediated (immediate) – some are caused by other parts of the immune system and are referred to as non-IgE mediated (delayed). We now know that these reactions are caused by different, slower-acting cells of the immune system. While the principle is the same – an inappropriate immune response to something that is actually harmless – an allergic reaction involving other parts of the immune system will look quite different due to the different chemicals released by the body.

The story of your child's reaction to food is very important in determining whether or not the reaction is IgE or non-IgE mediated. Allergy tests are also used to look for the presence and amount of IgE in your child's blood or skin and help to differentiate the different types of allergy.

If your child has an allergy, it doesn't mean that your child's immune system is weak. Food allergy is the result of a strong, but inappropriate, immune response to harmless food substances.

Why is the Correct Diagnosis Important?

It is important to distinguish between IgE and non-IgE mediated allergic responses because knowing the difference can change the management, and allow you to know the likely severity and the outcome of allergic disease for your child.

The good news is that the diagnosis of IgE mediated food allergy is much more straightforward once your child has had the allergy tests, as long as the results are properly interpreted to give a clear and thorough diagnosis of all the problem foods. At least at that point you know what you are dealing with!

The Allergic March

The allergic march is the name given to the progression through the different allergic or atopic illnesses that is commonly seen in children who have inherited atopic genes (see Chapter 10 for more detail). Atopic illnesses can be linked to family history, the environment and exposure. Children who have an allergic immune system often progress through these conditions from eczema to food allergy and then on to respiratory allergy, including asthma and allergic rhinitis, as they get older. Specific allergies are not inherited, only a tendency to allergic disease.

When my son Zach was little, I worried all the time about unknown and undiscovered allergies. I am allergic to all sorts of animals, so I assumed Zach might be, on top of his many food allergies. He is now three and a half and, as he has got older, I've realised that time will tell and I have learnt to relax more. As time passes, it's not that I worry less, but it's that Zach is more able to tell me how he feels and I therefore feel better able to manage any future allergies, than when he was a baby.

Babies who suffer from eczema are particularly at risk of having food allergies. The more severe the eczema and the earlier in life that it begins, the more likely there is to be a food allergy. A baby with severe eczema before three months of age is very likely to suffer from IgE mediated food allergies. Children with eczema and food allergy are also very likely to get later respiratory problems. For example, having egg allergy carries a 70 per cent risk of later asthma. The allergic march will be discussed throughout this book because understanding it is so important in the good management of a food-allergic child.

When talking to your child's allergy specialist, family history is important. Make sure that you know of *any* allergies, not just to food, on either side of the family. It doesn't mean that your child will also develop these allergies, but it can help to explain your child's symptoms, and it can give you and the allergist a guide to what to look out for in the future.

Outgrowing Different Food Allergies

Fortunately, it is possible to outgrow food allergies. It is not clear how this happens and there are few theories to explain it. The likelihood of outgrowing any food allergy is most closely related to the offending food.

With IgE mediated allergy, most children who are allergic to cow's milk and eggs outgrow the allergy. The allergic reaction can be mild or severe, depending on which proteins within the egg white or milk are being recognised by the immune system. Those with the milder form tend to outgrow the allergy in early childhood, often by age five, they have have a milder reaction and can also tolerate baked egg or milk. Children with the more severe form, where even baked allergen causes reactions, may not outgrow the allergy until their teenage years. A minority will remain allergic in adulthood. While allergy to wheat and soy are usually outgrown in early childhood, allergy to shellfish, fish, sesame and tree nuts are seldom outgrown. Around one in five children will outgrow a peanut allergy.

Studies have shown that children with milk, egg and peanut allergy who have small allergy tests at diagnosis seem to be more likely to outgrow these allergies, while the presence of other allergic problems such as asthma, allergic rhinitis or severe eczema make early outgrowing less likely. Ideally, repeating allergy tests and discussions with your doctor are the best ways to monitor your child's likelihood of outgrowing their allergies.

Delayed, non-IgE mediated allergy tends to be outgrown early and in most cases by the age of three. However, in more severe cases, especially with chronic gastrointestinal problems, they may persist for longer. Unfortunately, there is no value in repeated testing, so keeping a careful eye on the results of any accidental exposures, if there have been any, can help in deciding whether a trial of reintroduction would be worthwhile.

CHAPTER 2
Immediate Food Allergy Signs and Symptoms

When Zach was about two years old, I made a mistake and gave him a sip of cow's milk. Almost immediately, his lips and eyelids swelled and he started to itch his throat and nose. He developed red, itchy, blotchy hives on his chest and around his neck. I grabbed him, ran upstairs and gave him a big dose of Piriton. He got no worse and over the next 20 minutes or so the symptoms settled. That was his immediate reaction to cow's milk.

As you start to discover that your child has food allergies, you will become familiar with the signs and symptoms to look out for. General signs are covered in Chapter 6 but it is important to remember that many infants will suffer from stomach and bowel problems, incessant crying, poor sleep, restlessness, inability to self-soothe and faltering growth – all of which may not be related to food at all. It is important to know exactly how and when your child has reacted, because that will guide you and the healthcare professionals towards a formal diagnosis of food allergy. It is also important to be able to identify a severe reaction so that you can respond quickly.

In the previous chapter we discussed IgE (immediate) and non-IgE (delayed) mediated food allergy. These appear very differently so when discussing symptoms it is important to consider them separately. The way that these different types of allergy are diagnosed is also very different so you must try to be clear when you report the symptoms to the doctor so that he or she can differentiate between the two types and guide the investigations accordingly. We will discuss delayed reactions in more detail in the next chapter.

Mild to Moderate Symptoms
• •

IgE mediated allergies are relatively easy to spot. They happen suddenly with often striking symptoms and very quickly after the offending food has been eaten. This makes them easier to diagnose. Few parents who see their child develop hives within the first few minutes of their first bottle of formula or first exposure to peanut will not put two and two together. Where there is uncertainty about what food may have caused an allergic reaction then allergy testing can help to sort things out.

Mild to moderate symptoms of an immediate allergic reaction are a flushed face; hives; a red and an itchy rash around the mouth, tongue or eyes that can spread to the whole body; mild swelling of the lips, eyes and face; nausea and vomiting; tummy cramps and diarrhoea; a runny or blocked nose; sneezing and watery eyes. Although these symptoms are described as mild to moderate, as the parent of a baby or child who is suffering in this way, it can be frustrating, exhausting and concerning as you try to offer them comfort (see Chapter 7 which discusses everyday allergy management).

Severe symptoms (anaphylaxis) that require immediate medical attention are listed below. This type of severe reaction will be discussed further in Chapter 8.

- Throat tightness
- Wheezing
- Shortness of breath
- Repetitive coughing
- Difficulty breathing
- High-pitched noises when breathing
- Changes in voice or cry – hoarseness
- Turning pale or bluish

- Tongue swelling
- Difficulty swallowing
- Low blood pressure
- Fainting
- Chest pain
- Dizziness
- Feeling of impending doom (older children)

When a child with this type of food allergy accidentally eats or drinks what they are allergic to, it will cause symptoms almost straight away and usually within minutes. Reactions seldom occur more than 30 minutes after consumption and with this type of allergy, no more than two hours later. This can be a terrifying experience, but also one that can be managed well and safely with the appropriate treatment (see Chapter 8). Remember, if the food is hidden within another, for example a peanut in a chocolate bar, there may be a slight delay in symptoms occurring. Symptoms will usually focus on the area where there is contact, such as around the mouth, so swollen itchy lips and a rash on the face are very common. More serious and worrying symptoms include difficulty breathing or swallowing, skin colour changes and floppiness or drowsiness. Not every child will have every symptom. Each child will vary, and may even have different symptoms each time the same food or drink is consumed.

Reactions from contact with the skin, where the food is not consumed, will again be localised and are seldom more than just a rash. For example, a baby may come into contact with allergenic food when sat at an unclean high chair, or a toddler at nursery may come into contact with milk spilt by another child.

The different symptoms of food allergy occur because different organs and systems react in different ways when histamine is released by the body. There is no predictable order in which these symptoms occur. Your child may react with one symptom followed by another, or most likely, two or more symptoms in no predictable sequence. Generally, however, most reactions start around the mouth and end there too. Some may also involve tummy pain, vomiting, diarrhoea, itchy and watery eyes and an itchy nose. However, more severe reactions will spread rapidly and any sign of difficulty in breathing, a cough, change in voice (suggesting tightening of airway in the neck) should be treated as a medical emergency. Adrenaline (see page 119) must be given, if carried, and an ambulance called. Reactions where the blood pressure drops causing confusion and collapse or floppiness and drowsiness are more common when adults have severe reactions but may also happen in children.

The Common Food Allergens

The common food allergens are:

- Milk
- Egg
- Peanuts
- Tree nuts
- Wheat
- Soya
- Fish
- Shellfish
- Sesame seeds
- Kiwi fruit

Further symptoms

Eczema

There is a close link between eczema and food allergies. Babies who suffer from eczema are particularly at risk of food allergies, both delayed and immediate. Food allergies are more common in children from families where other members suffer from an allergy.

> *From 3 months old my daughter had bad eczema. I have forgotten how bad it was with the exception of one incident. One night during her sleep she scratched her face and took most of her skin off her cheeks and temples. There was a reasonable amount of blood on the sheets and my husband was away overseas at the time. It took a very long time to heal and she repeatedly scratched the healing scabs at every opportunity.*
>
> ANNE, MUM OF HANNAH AND EDWARD

Atopic dermatitis is a type of eczema, which is also referred to as allergic eczema. Throughout this book we will call it eczema. It is a dry, red and raw-looking rash that itches and can become infected if the skin becomes broken. If left untreated, it can cause skin damage, resulting in a blotchy appearance, which is especially noticeable in children with darker skin. It is estimated that atopic or allergic eczema now affects one in five children.

Often babies have skin symptoms, in addition to eczema, that are perfectly common, such as cradle cap and milk spots, and this can make diagnosis more difficult. Eczema, however, has a distinctive look. In infancy, it usually appears first on the face, then spreads elsewhere such as in creases of the legs and arms, at the ankle, behind the knee or elbow and can look like burn marks around the neck and the bottom. A characteristic of eczema is itching and you may notice your child itching when she is in the bath or when her clothes are removed, even before you can see any rash.

At about 3 months [my son's] eczema was really bad – someone described him as having crocodile skin. His skin was red and dry and horrible. He would tear himself apart if he could. Bath times were horrible times… I booked him into the allergy specialist and he was allergy tested at 4 months of age. By then I had done some reading and was starting to take foods out of my diet – egg and dairy first as they were two of the worst allergens (we were already nut-free due to my daughter's allergies). I was taking a detailed food diary and had made links to other foods… the results of his first allergy test were that he was allergic to dairy, egg, soy, wheat and nuts. I was advised to stop breastfeeding and give him elemental formula. His skin improved and for the first time he did not have diarrhoea (I did not even realise he did as he had always been like that).

ANNE, MUM OF HANNAH AND EDWARD

Eczema often occurs in babies and children who are predisposed to allergy, such as those who have relatives with eczema or other allergic problems such as asthma, hay fever or food allergies. The rash typically comes and goes, but can be triggered by skin irritants such as soap, sweating, clothing and detergents, or by infections, emotions such as stress or being upset, and allergies. As your child scratches their skin, it becomes inflamed and loses moisture.

The relationship between eczema and food allergy is complex. With IgE (immediate) type allergies, almost all children will have had at least some history of eczema. As mentioned earlier, having significant eczema during infancy is a major risk factor for IgE mediated food allergy and it is thought that this is not just a coincidence, but that the problems of having a leaky skin barrier, that is, skin that is irritated, broken down or infected, actually leads to the development of food allergies. Some studies in Japan have shown that aggressive treatment of eczema in babies may reduce the risk of food allergy developing. However, the relationship between food allergy and eczema is also seen during an allergic reaction, when eczema can flare up due to the body releasing histamine and this may lead to a more sustained period of the eczema being troublesome. There is also an important relationship between food allergy and eczema with delayed allergies, which is discussed in the next chapter.

Remember that even if you are breastfeeding, food proteins (e.g. milk and egg) in your diet will be passing via your breastmilk into your child's diet. In infants with an immediate type allergy to milk or egg, when this happens, rather than having an immediate type reaction, there may just be a worsening of eczema (similar to that seen in delayed food allergy). You should discuss this possibility with your doctor before trying to cut any foods out of your own diet. Without milk in your diet, you need to ensure you have an alternative source of calcium to make sure that your breast milk is providing enough calcium for the baby.

Eyes, ears, nose and throat

During an immediate allergic reaction, your child's eyes may become itchy, red and swollen. They may also develop a runny, itchy or blocked nose, sneezing, a sore throat and an itchy mouth and ears. Itchy ears are usually the result of the same nerves supplying both the palate and the ears, so histamine in the mouth due to contact with an allergenic food will cause a feeling of itchiness in the ears.

Stomach and bowel

Histamine released into the bowel due to an allergic reaction can lead to vomiting, stomach cramps and diarrhoea, all of sudden onset. These can be very unpleasant but are not necessarily signs of a severe, anaphylactic reaction.

Breathing problems

Specific breathing symptoms can occur as part of an allergic reaction. These include the sudden development of a blocked or runny nose, sneezing, an itchy nose and throat, coughing and tightening of the airways leading to asthma – difficulty in breathing and wheezing. Another important symptom is known as stridor, a harsh noise when your child breathes in (the same as that caused by croup), which is due to narrowing of the large airways in the neck. Like the asthma symptoms, stridor is a sign of anaphylaxis and needs emergency treatment with adrenaline and an ambulance to be called. Breathing problems are typical of a severe reaction in children, while adults having anaphylaxis tend to more commonly have confusion and collapse due to a drop in blood pressure (anaphylactic shock).

Eating or drinking the allergenic food protein is almost invariably the cause of a severe reaction to food, but inhaling can also trigger it. Such reactions are usually mild but can, less commonly, cause more troublesome symptoms of wheezing. Typically it is fish, usually being cooked, that is the most common culprit, although rarely other allergens such as milk can be aerosolised (for example, by coffee-making machines that froth milk) and cause problems. This is, however, very unusual and trying to avoid such scenarios can make life very difficult. The practical implications can be huge, as inhalation can occur when the food is being cooked or consumed such as in restaurants with open kitchens, or for airplane travel, where air is contained and recycled. It is worth discussing your concerns about your child having this type of reaction with your doctor. However, it may be that unless your child has reacted in this way, you as the parent just have to make a judgement call on avoidance of this situation. Bear in mind that this type of reaction is very rare.

It is worth noting that while breathing symptoms are sometimes part of an allergic reaction to food, they will almost invariably occur alongside the other typical features of hives, swelling and itching. Symptoms, such as a blocked nose, runny nose, sneezing or difficulty in breathing, in isolation of these other symptoms are extremely unlikely to be caused by food. They may be due to an allergy to airborne substances, such as pollen, or indeed other causes, such as regular asthma or infections.

CHAPTER 3
Delayed Food Allergy Signs and Symptoms

In the last chapter we discussed immediate, IgE mediated allergies, which are usually relatively easy to spot – rapid onset of rash and swelling around the mouth after a food is eaten. Such symptoms will often be recognised as an allergy by parent or doctor. However, more recently it has become apparent that our immune systems can react to food in other more subtle ways. Such non-IgE mediated reactions (so called as they don't involve the allergic antibody) may cause very troublesome symptoms but the lack of obvious and immediate reaction after the food is consumed can make them hard to spot and significant delay on diagnosis is common.

Non-IgE mediated allergies are often divided into very specific different conditions, which are discussed below, but there needs to be some context as children do not always fall in to specific patterns. In truth, delayed allergy is a spectrum of disease, in terms of its severity and where the problems show themselves such as in the gut or skin. It is therefore important to remember that many children will not fit one label easily.

Delayed, non-IgE mediated allergies do not happen straight after the food is eaten and there are no reliable allergy tests to help. This is compounded by a relative lack of knowledge and understanding about the part of the immune system that is involved. As a consequence, delayed allergies usually reveal themselves in a very different way to IgE allergies.

Most non-IgE mediated allergies appear during early infancy with the most common cause being cow's milk. Other causes include soya (often in those with a milk allergy too) and less so wheat and egg. It is very much milk that is the major allergen and the prime suspect whenever delayed allergy is suspected in infancy. Delayed allergies to other foods are much less common but can be severe (see FPIES, on page 31).

Typical symptoms of delayed allergies fall into two categories:

1. Skin
2. Stomach and bowel

Remember that, even though your child may be breastfed, allergens such as milk and soya can still get to him through the breast milk. Symptoms would usually be milder than if the child was eating or drinking the allergen directly. The relationship between the amount of allergen consumed and the symptoms is an important clue. If symptoms get much worse during the move from breastfeeding (when the only milk in your child's diet is what gets in via your diet) to bottle-feeding, then milk allergy needs careful consideration.

The Common Delayed Food Allergens

- Milk
- Egg
- Soya
- Wheat

Symptoms

Symptoms of a delayed allergic reaction include eczema, reflux, loose stools (although much less commonly constipation is possible), or persistent crying (often written off as colic). Less common but possibly related is faltering growth.

Skin

A typical symptom of delayed allergy is severe eczema that is indistinguishable from other eczema by sight alone. When the eczema is due to delayed food allergy, it is more likely to be severe as well as unresponsive to treatment such as moisturisers and steroid creams. As previously discussed, it is now widely recognised that children with severe, unresponsive eczema should always have food allergy considered.

Clues that your child's eczema may be related to diet include:

- Eczema that first appeared at less than six months of age.
- A family history of allergies such as asthma, eczema or hay fever.
- Eczema that doesn't respond as well as expected to treatment such as steroid creams.
- Stomach and bowel problems such as colic, reflux, diarrhoea or poor weight gain.
- Worsening of eczema after being breastfed or after meals, or generally worsening of eczema after transitioning from breast to bottle.
- The presence of one food allergy. If your child has an obvious allergy to one food, consider if another is also causing problems.

Levi had sensitive skin from birth really but from around five months old it started to get progressively worse. Rashes were all over his body especially his face and he was vomiting, had red itchy eyes and was sometimes wheezy. I visited my doctor and we were both convinced that allergies were to blame for the eczema... After seeing a paediatrician and a dermatologist, it emerged that Levi was allergic... The dermatologist realised that the bath oil he had been prescribed for his skin actually contained nut oil... The amazing thing was that as soon as we ceased using the oil and changed his milk, his skin recovered to almost perfect in a matter of about a week or two.

BEV, MUM OF LEVI

Stomach and bowel

Symptoms include reflux, colic, diarrhoea, poor weight gain, difficulty feeding and, less commonly, constipation. Your baby may simply scream all the time and back arch (often put down to 'silent' reflux). Remember that all of these symptoms are not uncommon in babies who do not have milk allergy, and hence separating those who do have an underlying allergy from those who don't is very challenging.

From birth to 12 weeks I saw three health visitors and four GPs, who all told me that S had colic and told me I was an anxious first-time mum. S was prescribed various medications from Gaviscon to lactulose, all of which exacerbated his digestive symptoms. My health visitor laughed when I said that S had such loud wind that it woke me up. However, I couldn't see what was so amusing when a baby screamed in pain as he passed wind. She also dismissed my desperate attempt to show her a nappy containing violent green diarrhoea seeking some explanation, stating that she had seen green poo before and didn't need to see it again; embarrassed, I hurriedly put the nappy to one side, once again feeling like a fussy amateur mum.

HANNAH, MUM OF S

Shortly after Charlie's six-week check things seemed to deteriorate. Charlie began to develop a runny nose and a really harsh-sounding cough and displayed colicky symptoms at around five every morning. Charlie's stools were also concerning me. At times they were very loose and bright yellow and at other times they would be an extremely dry stool and green in colour.

THANH, MUM OF CHARLIE

Again, like with eczema, clues include severity, resistance to treatment and the relationship with the amount of milk consumed (in other words, symptoms worsen when moving from breast to bottle). Another big clue that delayed allergy may be the cause of symptoms is the presence of both skin and bowel and stomach symptoms. Loose stools or reflux in the child with bad eczema; or troublesome eczema in the child with problematic reflux or colic should ring alarm bells.

Breathing problems

Breathing symptoms are a rarer problem in delayed allergy and as with immediate allergies do not happen in isolation of either skin or gut symptoms. Sometimes breathing symptoms such as noisy breathing or wheezing may occur due to reflux, where stomach contents spill over into the airway and hence there is an overlap.

For the two weeks following the introduction of formula milk, Charlie's wet-sounding wheezy cough did not improve, and he would still wake up with gas and abdominal pain. He was also still having hour-long coughing fits and so I went to see the GP to discuss the possibility of a cow's milk protein allergy and hopefully be prescribed a dairy-free formula.

THANH, MUM OF CHARLIE

Cow's Milk Protein-Induced Proctocolitis

This is a condition that babies get usually by the time they are two months old. It is part of the less harmful end of the spectrum of non-IgE mediated allergy to milk. Babies usually present with visible blood mixed with mucus in the stools. Finding blood in your baby's nappy is frightening and must always be investigated by your doctor as soon as possible. Otherwise they are well and thriving. It is more common in breastfed babies whose mothers are ingesting cow's milk or soya protein, although it can occur in babies on formula milk. The doctor may diagnose your baby with protocolitis having seen the positive response that your baby has to a period of excluding cow's milk protein from their diet, either by excluding it from the breastfeeding mother's diet or by giving the baby a hypoallergenic formula (see page 178). Bleeding should resolve in 72 hours. Diagnosis is confirmed by reintroducing the milk to see if the symptoms return.

What exactly is happening and why is unclear. However, children tend to outgrow it sooner than in IgE mediated milk allergy, with most tolerating cow's milk protein by one to two years of age. Milk reintroduction can be carried out safely by the parents or carers at home, although it is important that your doctor has ruled out an IgE mediated reaction first by a negative skin test result or specific IgE blood test.

Cow's Milk Protein-Induced Enteropathy

Unlike those with cow's milk protein-induced proctocolitis, children with enteropathy usually have long-standing diarrhoea and vomiting.

This can result in poor absorption, poor nutrition and faltering growth, making a firm diagnosis even more important. The development of your child's symptoms and their story will be similar to other forms of non-IgE mediated milk allergy, appearing in infancy and resolving by 1–2 years of age. Again, what exactly is happening in your child's body is unclear and blood and skin prick allergy tests are usually negative. The diagnosis is made after any infection is ruled out, through a combination of taking a sample of the tissue (biopsy) from your child's bowel and again the results of exclusion diets.

Food Protein-Induced Enterocolitis Syndrome (FPIES)

FPIES is a severe condition where your child's stomach and bowel become rapidly and severely inflamed, typically due to cow's milk or soy exposure. FPIES represents the severe end of the spectrum of milk allergy. It affects only the gut.

FPIES is characterised by severe protracted diarrhoea and vomiting, within a few hours of having cow's milk or soya-based formula (50 per cent of children affected react to both), although solid food allergens are occasionally implicated. The combination of vomiting and diarrhoea can result in dehydration and lethargy, often with the wrong diagnosis being made. Failing to recognise the link with your child's diet can result in multiple admissions to hospital with what is presumed to be recurrent severe infection.

Symptoms rapidly resolve on a diet free of allergens. Children with FPIES classically have negative allergy blood tests and negative results from skin prick testing. The diagnosis is made based on how your child is and negative allergy tests, with a cow's milk challenge (introducing cow's milk under medical supervision and monitoring your child's response) if doubt remains. Again, what exactly is happening in your child's body with FPIES is poorly understood.

Other Immune Mediated Reactions

Allergic Eosinophilic Gastroenteropathies are a group of conditions with overlapping symptoms, all characterised by swelling in the gut. They are classified according to the site of the swelling, although it is the depth and severity of the symptoms that will most influence how your child will appear. Again, what exactly is happening in the body remains uncertain but a diagnosis can only be made with a biopsy of the gut taken during an endoscopy (when a flexible tube is inserted in the mouth or anus to look at the gut internally).

Cow's milk protein-induced reflux oesophagitis

Although it is now clear that multiple food proteins may induce oesophagitis (swelling of the tube that leads from the throat to the stomach), the most common one is cow's milk protein. This variant of cow's milk allergy appears to be particularly common in children (up to 42 per cent of children with gastro-oesophageal reflux – GOR – disease), with symptoms identical to reflux but that settle on an exclusion diet. Many affected children have become sensitised to cow's milk protein, while exclusively breastfed. Again the underlying cause is unclear.

The best way to manage these allergies, as with immune mediated food allergy, is to avoid the offending allergen. In the case of milk allergy, especially as it is often the main source of nutrition in the children it affects, the involvement of a paediatric dietician is crucial. Informing parents about how to read food labels and avoid milk, as well as choose an appropriate substitute that ensures complete nutrition, requires considerable expertise. Further education on how to recognise and treat the reactions that may result from accidental exposure is also important. Regular follow-up appointments to monitor growth and the possible development of tolerance is also needed, as is a holistic approach to ensure recognition and treatment of other allergic conditions that these children so often have.

Diagnosis

A delayed allergy can only be diagnosed by showing that the symptoms get much better when the suspect allergen is removed and then return when it is introduced a few weeks later. Your doctor will need to take a careful history and decide if it is worth a trial elimination of the suspected allergen to clinch the diagnosis. Remember that allergy tests (which detect levels of IgE which are not relevant to non-IgE mediated reactions) are not helpful. There are national NICE (National Institute for Health and Care Excellence) guidelines for GPs that relate to the process of story-taking and diagnosis and there is a useful parents' guide to accompany this (please see the Resources section page 253).

CHAPTER 4
Allergy Testing

Identifying allergies accurately is essential for successful management. If the diagnosis is wrong, there is a risk of your child reacting to foods that aren't safe or instead safe food unnecessarily being excluded. The key to diagnosis is a good, allergy-focused history taken by an experienced healthcare professional. The important parts of this history are your child's story including her symptoms, their nature, how quickly they appear and how long they last. Together with details of a family and personal history of allergies, the doctor can make a decision as to whether food allergy is a likely cause. It can be useful to write this sort of information down so you have it to hand when you are asked.

If food allergy is suspected, then the doctor needs to decide which type of food allergy may be the issue – immediate (IgE mediated) (see page 4) or delayed (non-IgE mediated) (see page 5). Then investigations are required to confirm or exclude food as the cause. Which tests are carried out will depend very much on the suspected type of allergy. We will discuss the investigation of IgE and non-IgE mediated allergies separately to avoid confusion, although it is worth bearing in mind that some doctors may still be confused about this themselves. There is a real danger of misdiagnosis if tests intended for IgE mediated allergy are applied to children with suspected non-IgE mediated allergy and vice versa.

Tests for IgE Mediated Allergy
....

Essentials

- Levels of IgE in blood or skin tests alone are usually meaningless. They must be interpreted within the context of your child's story or they can lead to a confused diagnosis and unnecessary dietary elimination.

- There is no test to determine allergy severity. This depends on many factors that tests cannot predict.

- A supervised oral food challenge (see page 40) is considered the gold standard for food allergy testing, and can also be considered as a good way to 'rule out' food allergy.

By now, you may have begun to establish a pattern in your child's symptoms and their possible relationship to food. Remember typical IgE mediated reactions are rapid onset with hives, rash and swelling after food exposure, often the first or second time it has been consumed. In the UK, egg, milk, nuts, fish and shellfish are the most common causes. You have, most likely, begun weaning and have a repertoire of food that your child can eat and drink. After discussing your child's symptoms with your doctor, if IgE mediated allergy is suspected you will now have the chance for some formal allergy testing.

It is worth remembering that all of the weaning that you have done up until now is vital, as it is the best source of information for the doctors and dieticians to use, in combination with the allergy tests, to make a clear diagnosis. Allergy tests on their own are not reliable enough to confirm an allergy, but with a clear history of reactions or lack of them to food or drink, IgE mediated food allergies can be diagnosed quite readily. Remember your own diet may also be relevant if you are breastfeeding, due to the passage of food protein such as milk or egg, through your breast milk.

History alone is not enough to confirm food allergy, especially as allergies may be outgrown or the causative food may not have been obvious. Firm diagnosis requires testing. The skin prick tests and specific IgE blood test are only useful for immediate allergies. Unfortunately there are currently no useful tests for non-IgE mediated allergies.

What types of tests are available?

Blood and skin prick tests are best used to help confirm a suspicious history (your child having early onset eczema or reactions to food) for IgE mediated (immediate) food allergies. It is ideal if the tests are requested and interpreted by a specialist doctor so that specific foods, linked to your child's story can be tested for, and not just a range of different foods. This will help to minimise the amount of false positive results and will help to make the diagnosis clearer and minimise the consequent food allergy. The only reliable tests for an IgE mediated allergy are skin prick and specific IgE tests.

The gold standard for diagnosis of IgE (immediate) food allergy is a 'food challenge' where the suspected food is given to your child and your child is watched for signs and symptoms of an allergic reaction. Where IgE (immediate) allergy is suspected, a food 'challenge' (OFC) requires incremental feeding under observation for only a short period (see page 40). Unfortunately, a food challenge takes time and hospital resources and although it is safe when done properly, it still involves putting your child in harm's way. Allergy tests are therefore used to minimise the need for a food challenge, while still ensuring an accurate diagnosis. Sometimes there needs to be some compromise – for example, if a diagnosis is almost certain and it is felt a food challenge is not warranted to give absolute confirmation.

The severity of a future allergic reaction

Measurement of the size of the skin prick test wheal (see below) or the level of IgE in the blood helps to determine the likelihood of your child being allergic to a suspect food and must be interpreted in the context of your child's story. It is a common misconception among parents that the larger the size of the wheal or higher the level of IgE in the blood, the more severe an allergic reaction will be. This is not the case. There are no tests that can give an indication of the severity of an allergic reaction. The severity of an allergic reaction may depend upon a number of factors, such as the state of the allergen (cooked or raw) when it's eaten or the health of your child when she encounters the allergen or the amount of the allergen consumed. No test can predict these variables in advance. Below we go through the allergy tests in more detail.

Skin prick testing

Skin prick tests involve placing a drop of allergen on to the surface of the skin, and then pricking through the skin to introduce the allergen past the top layer. If IgE antibodies are present, then they will recognise the allergen and cause the release of a small amount of histamine – this produces an itchy bump and surrounding redness which should develop within 15 minutes. From a practical point of view, you will be asked to stop giving your child antihistamines prior to the skin prick tests taking place. You should stop long-acting antihistamines such as cetirizine (for example, Zirtek) and loratidine (for example, Clarityn) five days before the test and shorter-acting ones (for example, Piriton) two days before.

A negative skin prick test, where the skin shows no reaction is usually reliable at excluding allergy. However, a positive result, where there is a wheal and flare reaction (an itchy bump), can be indicative of allergy. The bump is measured and the bigger it is, the more likely it represents genuine allergy. These tests are not a reliable screening tool for diagnosis. They are useful, however, when screening for a specific allergen, related to a clear history of allergy that is consistent with an IgE mediated food allergy.

Specific IgE blood testing

This test (previously known as RAST test) measures levels of specific IgE for different foods in the blood. Mildly elevated results are often encountered, especially in children who have other types of allergic conditions such as eczema, asthma and allergic rhinitis. There is no need to stop giving your child antihistamines prior to having this blood test. Recently, a more sophisticated blood test called component testing has improved the diagnostic value of tests. While currently only used by specialists, this test looks at which part of the food is recognised by the immune system and can provide useful information about whether somebody is genuinely allergic or not.

The IgE blood test in isolation is a poor screening tool due to the high rates of falsely elevated and meaningless results. However, when carefully interpreted in the context of the clinical history, it can be very useful. It is also commonly misunderstood that higher IgE levels indicate increased 'severity'. Unfortunately, there is no test that can determine severity. Individuals with higher IgE results are at no more increased risk of anaphylaxis than someone with minimally positive tests, if they are indeed allergic at all. Like the skin prick tests, the higher the result, the more likely it represents genuine allergy but this must be interpreted in the context of your child's story.

Taking blood is always a pretty traumatic experience for both Zach and me. However, on all our visits, the hospital staff have been brilliant and caring. When they take blood, a play therapist entertains Zach, they show me how to hold him and they make sure he can't see the blood or needle.

Once it's over, we have lots of cuddles, a few soya chocolate buttons and he quickly stops crying. Local anaesthetic cream applied in advance can make things much less unpleasant.

Supervised oral food challenge

The oral food challenge is considered the gold standard for food allergy testing. It involves eating or drinking gradually increasing amounts of the suspected food allergen while being supervised by a doctor or nurse, usually an allergist. If your child does not react, then it is considered that there is no allergy to that food. Before a food challenge, symptoms must be under control and the suspected allergenic food not eaten for 7–14 days and antihistamine medication stopped. Most food challenges are done when it is suspected that somebody with a known allergy has outgrown it, suggested by a drop in the level of specific IgE in the blood test or size of the wheal in the skin prick test over time. Sometimes, but less often, a challenge is needed to make an initial allergic diagnosis, usually because there is a discrepancy between the allergy test and the child's story.

While the tests are not definitive, it is generally accepted that skin or blood tests or both, combined with a clear story, can confirm the presence of allergy in most cases and thus mean that a food challenge is not required. However, this approach will occasionally lead to over-diagnosis. For example, parents wrongly told that their children are allergic to things that they are not.

We had a baked egg challenge when Zach was aged two-and-a-half. The hospital staff began by giving him a tiny crumb of cake and then increasing the amount every 15 minutes. We did well and got through about a quarter of a cupcake, but then Zach reacted badly. Surprisingly, I felt incredibly safe. The doctors and nurses were on hand and dealt with the reaction immediately. I was looked after and allowed to just cuddle Zach through the experience. While I wouldn't want to go through it again, it was a well-managed, overall almost positive experience for both Zach and me.

Non-IgE mediated allergy

Unfortunately, the blood and skin tests are only for the diagnosis of IgE mediated allergies and are not useful for delayed allergies. Likewise, tests often available on the internet such as hair analysis, kinesiology, VEGA testing or IgG testing have no scientific evidence to support their value. The only useful test for non-IgE mediated allergy is the exclusion and reintroduction diet.

Classically, symptoms of delayed allergies, such as eczema or stomach and bowel symptoms cause persistent problems. A careful history of your child taken by the doctor will explore the possibility that these symptoms are due to food, the most common scenario being an allergy to cow's milk during infancy, and he or she will decide whether a trial exclusion is warranted. If so, this should really only be done under the supervision of a dietician as there is a risk of nutritional deficiency if it is not expertly handled, especially in small babies. Completely cutting out the suspected allergen should lead to a marked improvement in your child within one to two weeks. The diagnosis is not complete until reintroduction. If your child's symptoms return at this point, you can be confident that there is a delayed allergy and plans can be made to exclude the food, again with dietetic support.

CHAPTER 5
Your Allergy Clinic Appointment

Essentials

- Allergy testing is only part of the story.
- A good allergy clinic visit involves a detailed history, allergy testing and a clear management plan, as well as involvement of a dietician.

The first port of call for any person worried about food allergy is the GP. A GP can be a wonderful, supportive, knowledgeable resource in the community and it is from this start that your journey towards diagnosis and referring to specialists begins. Discuss your worries with your health visitor as well because postnatal care is routine and generally very well set up. The health visitor may have experience or advice that she can share with you.

Healthcare Professionals – Who's Who?

General practitioner – your general doctor and first port of call.

Health visitor – often will see you and your baby most frequently. Able to liaise with other healthcare professionals and help with advice and support.

Paediatrician – consultant who specialises in children.

Paediatric allergist – consultant who specialises in childhood allergy.

Dermatologist – consultant who specialises in skin conditions.

Immunologist – consultant who specialises in all aspects of the immune system.

Consultant in respiratory medicine – consultant who specialises in breathing conditions.

Dietician – an allied health professional who specialises in diet and nutrition. There are paediatric allergy dieticians who are children's dieticians with a special interest and experience in managing allergy.

Nurse specialists – nurses who have most experience and expertise within a certain field such as allergy or dermatology.

Play specialists – professionals who specialise in communicating with and helping children through play. They are often in hospital to help your child with many aspects of illness including allergy.

The clinic

In terms of allergies, every child needs to be assessed as an individual. It is difficult to generalise about what to expect from your doctor because your individual child and their unique circumstances are so important. However, there are a few lines of assessment that you can expect to be followed, which can be used to guide you through what to expect from your child's doctor. These are defined in the National Institute for Health and Care Excellence (NICE, 2011), which has an excellent guide for parents available from the www.nice.org.uk website.

Your child's 'story'

When your child is seen in the clinic, the first and most important thing is that the doctor takes a detailed, personalised story and gets an idea of the context of your child and family. This is also the most important part of the diagnostic process. You should be asked about other allergies, other family members and your child's symptoms – their nature, duration and relationship to possible triggers, as well as any other previous or ongoing medical issues. There should be discussion of how these are affecting both your child and the family in terms of their impact on quality of life. This is called an allergy-focused clinical history, which experts agree is the best way to assess a child and family for allergies and their management when they first meet the doctor (NICE guidelines, 2011).

The next stage is to listen again to the story and the symptoms to try to work out the allergic source, if any. There may only be subtle clues from each symptom to be pieced together. So, for each symptom, whether it be colic, reflux, tummy pain or more clear symptoms of allergy such as hives or swelling, thought needs to be given as to whether food allergy is likely and if so, what allergen is the most likely and what type of allergy it might be. As discussed earlier, allergies are usually broadly categorised into two groups – the immediate reactions (IgE mediated) and the delayed (non-IgE mediated).

Carrying out tests

For suspected immediate reactions (see page 4), allergy tests should be carried out. Ideally, skin prick tests are carried out there and then in clinic. You may well have been asked to avoid giving your child any antihistamines for five days before the appointment, otherwise these can get in the way of the test. Skin prick tests may be carried out by a nurse or the doctor and provide almost immediate and, in the right context, accurate results, which can then be discussed and a formal diagnosis made.

Sometimes, the combination of your child's story and skin test do not give quite enough information and it may also be necessary to carry out blood tests. One test is not better than the other and some clinics may only offer blood tests. The main downside (apart from the needle involved!) is that the results are not immediate, as they need to be sent to a lab for analysis.

It is important to know that these tests are reliable if interpreted carefully in the light of the story, even in young children. Some parents are inaccurately told that there is no worth in these tests as their baby is young and has a changing and maturing immune system. The tests *are* valid and useful but the key is having a qualified allergy doctor to interpret the results. As with any medical test, its worth is only as good as the person who interprets it. On their own, they have little value, but with your child's story and clinical picture (the way their symptoms seem to be appearing), skin prick and blood tests are an invaluable source of accurate information that often leads to a definite diagnosis. If this combination is not enough to reach a diagnosis, then a food challenge, where the child is carefully exposed to a suspect food under medical supervision, may be required (see page 40).

If the second group of symptoms, delayed allergic reaction (see page 5), is suspected, the only way to confirm is to try a period of food elimination and then reintroduce that food with supervision and look at the results. Allergy testing is seldom useful in this context.

Allergy test results need to be discussed with your doctor and firm decisions reached about what foods your child needs to avoid and which are safe. Further testing may be required to make these decisions.

Having a clear diagnosis is important, but it is not the whole story. You will need to know how to deal with food avoidance, about weaning and how to ensure that your child is getting adequate nutrition despite the restrictions. This means a further discussion is required and may well be led by a paediatric dietician in the clinic. Most large, specialist clinics will offer this during the visit, while others may need to refer you on for this on another day. Either way it is essential that it happens. Sending you off to manage a new allergy without such advice is not really good enough. You need to know how to read food labels, how to deal with 'may contain' labels, to know the common foods you will need to avoid and how to make up for any nutrients that are going to be otherwise missed out. If you aren't offered an appointment with a dietician, ask for one. The NICE guidelines (see page 45) are clear that you should have this.

An emergency plan

Written information is also important, including an emergency plan, especially if your child has an immediate type allergy. Make sure that you are clear about exactly what to do in case of a reaction occurring and that this information is available for your child's nursery, preschool and school. This may involve a discussion of whether it is necessary to carry adrenaline due to an increased risk of severe reactions. You may also want a 'travel plan' – a letter for airline security, especially if you are going to be carrying adrenaline autoinjectors. You can also ask about other precautions, such as medic alert bracelets. In addition, you should also be provided details of appropriate support groups such as Allergy UK or the Anaphylaxis Campaign (see page 258). Also try to discuss any psychological issues that your child's new diagnosis may bring up, as these may be addressed further by an appropriate expert. Feeding issues such as fussy eating or food refusal are more common in children with food allergy and the input of a dietician, feeding clinic or psychologist may be useful here. A final topic to discuss is follow-up.

Follow-up appointments

There is no correct time to follow up a child with allergies – this is very individual. If your child has just been diagnosed with multiple food allergies, or if the diagnostic process is not complete, then it may be appropriate to be seen just a few weeks after the first appointment. For children who are settled with a clear diagnosis, it may not be necessary to be seen more often than every few years, especially if they have an allergy that is unlikely to be outgrown.

Every child's circumstances are slightly different but so are the circumstances of the clinic you attend and busier clinics will have less space to see you often. Many children are seen by a local general paediatric clinic more regularly while attending the more specialist allergy clinic only every few years. To help increase capacity for regular reviews due to overwhelming demand, allergy clinics are being set up in community and health centres, which are run by dieticians and nurse specialists. These are set up around the bigger specialist allergy centres so far but are a model of care that may be used nationally in order to meet demand and give you and your child improved access to allergy services.

Reasons for a follow-up appointment include repeat testing for tolerance as fortunately many allergies are outgrown, especially milk, egg, wheat and soy (both delayed and immediate), while reactions to nuts, fish and shellfish are less commonly so. Repeating allergy tests and comparing them to previous tests is a useful way to see if something is changing and 'tolerance' is being developed. The decision as to whether it is worth trying a food again, as tolerance is suspected, will be based on allergy tests as well as any recent history of exposure, together with knowledge of what tends to happen with that particular allergy.

The timing of a review appointment in the allergy clinic will also depend on the age of your child and his chance of outgrowing his allergies. For example, a child who in a food trial can tolerate baked milk, for example in a cupcake, is likely to outgrow a milk allergy in early childhood, so a review during early childhood would be recommended. Whereas children who cannot tolerate baked milk are more likely to outgrow their milk allergy in later childhood, so should be reviewed when they are older. However, there are also other indicators. Whether an attempted reintroduction of the offending allergen takes place under hospital supervision or at home is something that should be discussed with your doctor.

Another reason for follow-up is to go through a revision of education around managing the allergy. The use of adrenaline autoinjectors (see page 118) and family management of severe allergic reaction should be reviewed yearly to ensure safety, as the first-aid procedures can be quickly forgotten if not regularly reviewed. This can be managed in community clinics, or by the nurse specialist. It is also important to have a regular dietetic review, especially in younger children with multiple allergies.

A further reason for follow-up is to review other allergic issues that so often go hand in hand with the food allergy, such as eczema as well as asthma or allergic rhinitis. Poorly controlled asthma increases the risk of severe reactions. Detecting a new diagnosis of asthma in a child with food allergy may mean a change in the emergency management plan, such that adrenaline needs to be carried. Allergic rhinitis can make asthma worse, which again can make food allergic reactions worse still. The different allergic conditions overlap and are linked, and therefore your child needs to be monitored closely for any signs of symptom progression or new symptoms. This way management of the allergy can be the best it should be at all times. We will discuss what is known as the 'allergic march' in more detail in Chapter 10. If there are ongoing issues with eczema or asthma, you may also be reviewed in a different clinic (such as dermatology or general paediatrics) alongside the allergy reviews. It is important that the clinics know who else you are seeing so that they can copy the relevant people in on any clinic correspondence.

Your experiences

The journey to your child being diagnosed with a food allergy may not have been smooth. In the UK, the GP is the first port of call and can be a brilliant source of information and support. However, a GP may not always immediately link the seemingly innocuous symptoms like colic, tummy ache, diarrhoea or reflux with food allergy. Medical knowledge is advancing all the time but as the period of time spent at medical school remains the same, the time available for gaining knowledge about allergies may well be limited. Persevere, however, and keep going back to the GP when symptoms don't improve or in fact deteriorate further. A very useful resource for parents is the NICE parent guide, *Food Allergy in Children and Young People*, (www.nice.org.uk). Your GP will also have a copy at the practice of the NICE guidelines for healthcare professionals (2011). Both of these documents provide clear guidance and assessment tools to help you as the parent, together with the GP, to come to the correct diagnosis and refer your child on to the right management path for his allergies.

> *I have learnt to fight for S with doctors/hospitals etc. as unfortunately this has been my experience. It is very strange because as a health professional myself I never liked 'he who shouts loudest', however I have found that unless you push to be heard you don't find the support. Insisting on a dietician is vital as they are the experts and will support you through this very challenging process.*
>
> HANNAH, MUM OF S

Diagnosing a Food Allergy
∙∙∙

The National Institute for Health and Care Excellence states in the food allergy guidelines that correct diagnosis is essential to reduce the incidence of adverse reactions to food and the number of unnecessary diets (www.nice.org.uk). Sometimes food allergies can be subtle and difficult to detect, especially delayed allergies, which tend to be a problem in infancy. Working out whether the problem is a food allergy can be very difficult and requires the help of an experienced doctor.

At four-and-a-half months, in desperation, my husband tried to give Alex a bottle of formula in an attempt to get him to sleep for longer than 30 minutes. His screaming only got louder, in what we thought was frustration at being given a bottle and so we never tried it again.

At five months the screaming became constant and I presented the two of us at A&E desperate for them to 'fix' him. His crying was so intense that they started investigations for meningitis and my little baby had a lumbar puncture and a CT scan (both thankfully clear). I spent two days on the ward pacing with a screaming, inconsolable baby, with the nurses trying to get me to give him a bottle but me, somehow, knowing that wasn't going to be the answer.

Then a lovely paediatrician appeared and gently suggested that he might be allergic to cow's milk. I told her not to be ridiculous as he wasn't even weaned, and she pointed out that the dairy proteins can cross into breast milk and all the 'comfort' biscuits I had been eating might not have been helping! I was again dismissive telling her I didn't really 'believe' in intolerances (don't get me wrong, I believe in allergy but equated 'intolerance' with people who were simply being a bit precious!) but, in desperation I agreed to try going dairy-free to allow his digestive system time to recover from the possible allergic reaction. I saw the dietician who gave me some really useful sheets and some calcium supplements. Alex was prescribed CMP-free [cow's milk protein-free] formula in case I found dairy-free too difficult. We did try that formula a couple of times but he screamed and screamed and so we abandoned it completely. I wish I could say I embraced healthy, dairy-free living, but I mainly spent the next four months eating bourbons and hobnobs!

Weaning him was a bit of a challenge as I didn't want to expose him to soya so had to express the milk he needed for his cereal, but he did well on this plus fruit and veg for a few months. It was at this time I went back to work and he breastfed in the mornings and then had no milk at all until I collected him. He then fed a great deal at night!

Gradually he did seem to become less unsettled and within a month was no longer screaming in pain or being sick all the time. By a year old we started to reintroduce CMP – first into my diet and then giving him some directly, and it was a great success. Now at 5 he eats a full diet and the whole thing is starting to become a distant memory.

SAM, MUM OF ALEX

As we have established already, diagnosing a food allergy is unfortunately more complicated than a single test and therefore your account of what happens and has happened to your child is the most important part of the diagnostic process.

It is so important that you, your GP, allergist, dietician and paediatrician all work together to understand what is happening and why it is happening to your child in order to help them the most.

During our first appointment with the paediatrician, I breastfed Zach and she was able to watch the process, the urgency with which he fed and then the squirming distressed baby that he became and how he would pull away from me and cry. She said that she would refer him to a hospital-based paediatrician who specialises in allergy and speak to a dietician about a non-allergenic formula. I felt that we had had a breakthrough. I felt redeemed almost, that I wasn't going mad, I wasn't just sleep deprived but there was something very wrong and that it needed to be investigated. The letter of referral that she wrote described Zach as 'a little boy under a lot of stress'. It was awful to read, but absolutely correct.

Monitoring Food and Symptoms

While food diaries can become a bit confusing and are not recommended in the NICE guidance, keeping a record of symptoms and dividing these into immediate and delayed type is a good approach.

For immediate type allergies, the doctor will want to know what the symptoms are, how rapidly they came and went, what food was eaten just beforehand and what treatment was given. If your child has ongoing symptoms and delayed allergy is suspected, it is useful to have a two-week diary of symptoms along with a record of the food eaten. These symptoms include any rashes, stools, episodes of colic or reflux and other illness. However, it is important that you don't spend time trying to connect symptoms with the food eaten. It doesn't necessarily work with chronic symptoms and requires considerable expertise to work out the suspect foods. Allergic symptoms that are mild, such as rashes, come and go and can take a few days to develop after eating the food. This means there is a real chance that making assumptions can make things very confused. It is important that you keep an open mind and try to keep tabs on the symptoms, in order to get a clear picture of what may be happening. Once your child has been seen by a doctor and dietician, it may be recommended that a food such as cow's milk be eliminated from the diet. At this point it may be worth repeating the symptoms diary for another two-week period to monitor any changes and again repeat when the food is reintroduced to your child's diet. This will allow an objective decision to be made as to whether the elimination has made any difference to your child. The eliminations and reintroductions of food *must be* carried out under the supervision of a dietician.

As already discussed, try to keep a diary for up to two weeks and then repeat it again if your child's diet changes under supervision, particularly if this is an important allergen such as milk, soy or wheat. If at all unsure, keep food labels as well so that your doctor or dietician can go through these looking for the culprit allergens. Ready-made and processed food can contain different ingredients so, for example, one fishfinger is not the same as another from a different manufacturer. Ingredients can change as well, so always check food labels. Include any medication that your child has had and any reactions within that period. If your child is at nursery, or with a childminder, those carers also need to be involved and fill out the charts as well. Write down any symptoms, no matter how unrelated they appear to be. Also monitor disturbances in sleep, unsettled behaviour and crying.

Before we had a confirmed diagnosis for Zach, we went through a whole load of suggestions and ideas about why he was so unsettled. These ranged from hunger and teething, to being a boy and being intelligent. We just didn't have a clue.

Symptom diary for suspected IgE mediated allergies

What are the symptoms?	How rapidly did they come and go?	What food was eaten just beforehand? (include major allergens, such as peanuts, tree nuts, milk, egg, wheat, soya, fish, shellfish, sesame, kiwi fruit)	What treatment was given?

As we have discussed, the gold standard test for diagnosis of a delayed allergy requires a complete exclusion of the suspect food or drink for a period of 2–8 weeks followed by reintroduction. As milk is the most common, this is the example that we have used in the diaries that follow and in the explanation of those diaries. To be certain that milk allergy is a problem, an improvement in symptoms should be seen when milk is excluded followed by a return of the symptoms on reintroduction.

The diaries allow the recording of symptoms for later comparison. It is done in three phases:

Pre-milk exclusion: Recording of symptoms for a one-week period prior to milk exclusion. This provides a baseline for comparison.

During milk exclusion: Recording of symptoms for a two-week period after milk exclusion has been fully implemented. It is recommended that you do not record the symptoms until two weeks after starting the exclusion diet as commonly there is some residual milk left in the diet for a few days.

Post-reintroduction: Recording of symptoms for a one-week period after milk is fully reintroduced to see whether symptoms return.

Completing the diary

The suggested symptoms are those commonly caused by milk allergy but the most important ones are those that your child has been suffering from. Many children with milk allergy have symptoms in just one area such as the skin, but have no gut problems at all, so you only need to complete the entries that relate to your child. Remember that the important thing is to be able to compare symptoms before, during and after the exclusion diet so, for example, with eczema, use a score of 0 to 5 to grade how bad the eczema is and stick to the same system throughout. For stool frequency or reflux, it may be easier to stick to the number of episodes that happen each day. Discuss how you are going to fill this diary in with your doctor or dietician and then discuss your findings with them.

Week 0 – Before Milk Exclusion

Symptoms	Day 1	Day 2	Day 3	Day 4	Day 5	Day 6	Day 7
Eczema severity Scale 0–5							
Stools passed							
Stool consistency							
Mucus in stools							
Night-time waking							
Appetite							
Episodes of reflux							
Other							
Other							

Week 1 – During Milk Exclusion

Symptoms	Day 1	Day 2	Day 3	Day 4	Day 5	Day 6	Day 7
Eczema severity Scale 0–5							
Stools passed							
Stool consistency							
Mucus in stools							
Night-time waking							
Appetite							
Episodes of reflux							
Other							
Other							

Week 2 – During Milk Exclusion

Symptoms	Day 1	Day 2	Day 3	Day 4	Day 5	Day 6	Day 7
Eczema severity Scale 0–5							
Stools passed							
Stool consistency							
Mucus in stools							
Night-time waking							
Appetite							
Episodes of reflux							
Other							
Other							

Milk Fully Reintroduced

Symptoms	Day 1	Day 2	Day 3	Day 4	Day 5	Day 6	Day 7
Eczema severity Scale 0–5							
Stools passed							
Stool consistency							
Mucus in stools							
Night-time waking							
Appetite							
Episodes of reflux							
Other							
Other							

Your child's story is the key to diagnosis, so try to be clear, despite your exhaustion, about the symptoms, triggers and duration. Remember to write down any questions that you have before your appointment with the doctor and dietician. Take photos of rashes in case your child hasn't got the rash when you see the doctor. When your appointment has finished, always ask for the details of who to contact when further questions, which you will inevitably have, come up in the future.

What Will Your Doctor Do?

Zach's paediatrician was wonderful and a few days after our appointment she phoned me with the name of a formula, Neocate. She had also referred us to a dermatologist, dietician and paediatric allergy specialist. The paediatrician also made another referral to a specialist for suspected gastro-oesophageal reflux thought to be associated with the difficulty feeding and sleeping. I was so grateful and relieved, I cried.

> *The consultant who we saw when Felix was nine months old was amazing. She completely confirmed all our thoughts, which was a huge relief. But up until then we didn't have clear answers from any health professionals and it felt for a long time like we were making things up. At one point I wondered if I would be breastfeeding forever as I didn't dare try any formula!*
>
> EMILY, MUM OF FELIX

Many of the healthcare professionals that you see can refer your child for allergy testing and begin the process of diagnosing and managing your child's symptoms. It is very important that you feel that the professionals are listening to you, explaining things to you and that lifestyle and circumstances are part and parcel of the management plan that is decided upon.

> *When visiting doctors I believe that seeing a specialist is key. I have heard so much mixed information and advice that other medical professionals give to people that leads me to believe that only an allergist will do. When you get to the allergist always write down everything you want to cover while there – questions, worries etc. This is so important as you will regret missing something.*
>
> BEV, MUM OF LEVI

CHAPTER 6
The Early Days with an Allergic Child

Food allergy, particularly the delayed type, can affect babies and children in a wide variety of ways. The physical symptoms vary hugely. Your child may have a bloated stomach, suffer from chronic or constant gas, be sick frequently and cry incessantly. She may vomit after eating and have constipation or diarrhoea. She may have disturbed sleep from the itchiness of eczema or the pain of trapped wind and seem to be unable to be calm by herself, needing almost constant attention from you, the parent. Your child may also eat a lot, mistaking the pains of flatulence for the pangs of hunger, or she may refuse to eat at all, resulting in faltering growth. Additionally, your child may also be at risk of poor nutrition.

Quick identification, correct diagnosis and an optimal management plan are therefore very important in order to minimise the physical as well as the social and behavioural aspects of food allergy. If you feel that your child is not improving with her current management plan, it is vital to ensure that you receive better management through correct diagnosis. If, for example, your child is being managed by a GP yet she is not improving, now may be the right time to ask for a referral to a paediatrician for ongoing care. This chapter goes through some of the symptoms and behaviours that you may be experiencing with your allergic child.

Common symptoms

Colic

It is not clear what the link is between food allergy and colic and results of studies looking at the link between colic and diet have been varied. In some cases, colic (essentially, persistent crying) can be due to underlying food (particularly cow's milk) allergy, yet most colic is not. Its causes are unknown and although it goes away, there are no proven effective treatments. Interestingly in cultures where babies are swaddled on their mothers, colic is very rare. Clues that colic may be related to food allergy are when it starts very early in infancy, the baby can't be consoled and it fails to get better. Worsening colic when the baby moves from being breastfed to bottle-fed or the presence of other potentially allergic symptoms, such as eczema or loose stools, should also raise the possibility of milk allergy. Therefore, if colic is a major issue for your baby, it may be of benefit to remove cow's milk from her diet or from that of the breastfeeding mother. This should only be undertaken with the support and advice from your GP or dietician.

From birth, S was a very unsettled newborn who could cry from when he woke up through to when he fell asleep. His cry was very loud and high-pitched and I realised that other babies didn't cry like him. He cried as if he was in pain. My health visitor and GP said he had colic and to sit it out, reassuring me he would improve after three months. When he was 12 weeks his insides were so raw from his allergies that he had a gastro-intestinal bleed. His nappy was full of blood and he continued to have bloody nappies for the rest of the day. We took him to the children's hospital and the doctors suggested that he had a milk allergy. As I was breastfeeding him they suggested that I came off dairy for a week and see what happened to his symptoms. Within two days S turned into a very content smiley little baby who rarely cried – the difference was astonishing.

HANNAH, MUM OF S

Crying, distress and sleep disturbance

Zach was a very distressed, highly alert and unsettled small baby. He fed and cried endlessly and slept for short periods of time, often just 45 minutes day and night. He was really sensitive to noise and really jumpy so would wake as soon as he fell asleep.

The discomfort that your baby may be feeling due to the incessant itching from their skin, or from their bowel problems, combined with reflux and colic is a concoction that will inevitably lead to your baby's sleep being disturbed. When she is young and learning how to self-soothe at night-time, the physical symptoms that your baby is experiencing will make the process of achieving a relatively restful night a particular challenge. As with all babies, establishing a bedtime routine is important. The nightly skincare routine should be rigidly followed and the bedroom should be kept cool, with mitts being used at night-time. Some parents may try tilting the bed to help with the reflux and others offer comforters such as dummies to help through phases of particularly poor sleep. It is important to not worry too much at this time about what the baby books say in terms of hours of sleep, ability to self-soothe and even leaving your baby to cry it out. Remember that your baby has challenges of her own which will not be addressed in baby books and which your other friends' babies may not be experiencing. Therefore, it is advisable to respond to your baby and try whatever works for you and your child to achieve maximum rest and peace, especially at night.

Like clockwork, he would draw his legs up at around 5am every morning and scream in pain. His sleep had also gotten progressively worse and I had resorted to breastfeeding him all night, as it seemed to be the only thing that would soothe him. I remember feeling like I was creating a vicious circle as this probably added to his gassiness.

THANH, MUM OF CHARLIE

Remember not to just put up with this. If your baby has ongoing symptoms affecting her sleep, discuss these with your doctor. It may be due to something in your or her diet, or it may mean medication is required for the eczema or gastrointestinal symptoms. However, it is also important to recognise that symptoms can sometimes not be due to the allergies, even if your baby has them. A child with an egg allergy, who is completely egg free, may still get eczema or reflux that is difficult to control but unrelated to the rest of their diet.

It can be easy for parents to sometimes assume that everything is due to something in the diet and this can lead to difficult and unnecessary overly restrictive diets.

Feeding issues

Babies with gastrointestinal symptoms may be hungrier, as they are not absorbing the nutrients from the milk that they are being given. These babies will therefore feed more frequently. Babies who are allergic, may feed more frequently as a form of gaining comfort. If you are breastfeeding your baby, it may be the case that your baby develops symptoms from allergens in your breast milk. This can make the experience of breastfeeding a difficult and distressing one for both your baby and you. Your baby is desperate to feed but then becomes quickly distressed when she does as the symptoms of allergy become exacerbated. She may desperately try to latch on to your breast and then suddenly pull off. Your baby may be so exhausted from the symptoms and poor sleep that it's a struggle to keep her awake to achieve a full feed when she starts to breastfeed. As a mum, you are trying to feed your distressed baby, who may be writhing around in discomfort, scratching as she begins to react to allergens in your milk but then trying to latch on again for comfort.

If you are breastfeeding your baby, it is really important to look after yourself and get some help. Even though your baby is reacting in the way that she is because of her symptoms, the results can be the same as for someone who is having difficulty breastfeeding in the first place. To help you to hold your baby correctly to feed, anticipate her movements, protect your nipples from becoming sore and ultimately prevent a poor breastfeeding technique, seek help from your health visitor. Try to have the confidence, no matter how you may feel, to ask for help repeatedly if necessary, to allow the health visitor to watch you feed and to help you. Try, if you can, to establish a feeding routine, based on how often your baby should be feeding and on how hungry your baby seems. Time how long each feed is for and try to offer both breasts at each feed so that you can learn what a sufficient feed is for your baby. Expressing your breast milk, in order to measure it and giving it in a bottle is also another way to monitor your baby's intake of milk. If you can, try to share the feeding with your partner to take the strain off you and share the difficulties and joys of feeding your baby. There are organisations that are set up to help breastfeeding mothers and it may be that they can put you in touch with someone who can help if they are unable to. Either way, it is important to seek professional help and advice. There are links in the Resources section at the back of this book (see page 254), which may be of use to you.

Charlie's daytime feeding had started to get worse as well. He would seem really desperate to feed but when he latched on he would pull off and cry. I started to become extremely frustrated and, coupled with the sleep deprivation things got really bad for our family... On reflection, Charlie's feeding patterns both with exclusive breastfeeding and weaning onto solids were what eventually led me to suspect that Charlie had a cow's milk protein allergy. Once breastfeeding was fully established, he would only stay on the breast for about ten minutes and very rarely would he take both breasts. I thought that he may just be a very efficient feeder and was told that was probably the case by the health visitor. I did notice that he was slowly shifting centiles and was not gaining much weight, which I raised with the GP and the nursery nurses and the health visitors at the clinic.

I was physically and emotionally exhausted. I didn't understand why he would not sleep for longer than a two-hour period and why weaning him on to solid food was so difficult... Charlie has since been prescribed amino acid formula by our GP and we have not looked back. My baby is finally gaining weight as he should be and is approaching the twenty-fifth centile having dropped to the second. He is sleeping better, no longer having coughing fits or bouts of colic...

THANH, MUM OF CHARLIE

Despite its challenges, breast milk remains the best food for your baby, especially in the first six months of life and while excluding certain foods from your diet can be difficult, it can be worth it if it means your baby stays breastfed. However, if a baby has multiple allergies (and you are having to exclude multiple foods from your diet) there may occasionally be circumstances when breastfeeding stops being viable. This is something you should discuss with your doctor or dietician. Stopping breastfeeding can be upsetting but sometimes it is the best option for both you and your baby.

While there are a lot of good support networks available online, it is important to remember that there is a lot of well-intentioned, misinformation available. Someone else's experience may be irrelevant or even harmful to yours. Allergy UK (+44 1322 619898) and the Anaphylaxis Campaign (+44 1252 542029) have helpline telephone numbers where professionals can provide you with a wealth of practical support and advice, as well as information about support groups in your local area.

Impact on the Family

It can be difficult for the rest of your family to understand exactly what is going on with your baby. You may find that family members have all sorts of suggestions and solutions, some of which may be useful and some of which may not be. A child with allergies has an impact on the whole family, not just on you as the parent and it is important to try to recognise that impact and involve the wider family from early on, if possible. Even if you can find one member of your extended family who you can talk to, who will listen and understand, that can be so helpful to both you and them in terms of understanding and being able to give you the support you need. If your extended family do not understand what is happening, they will not be able to help you.

Of course, there will be those who refuse to listen and empathise and you will need to decide how to deal with that. Often with time, people learn more and come to understand and accept the situation. However, that delay can be emotional and stressful for you. Try to be patient with relatives and, in the meantime, accept that childcare from those people is just not an option and focus your energies elsewhere. Remember that grandparents often struggle with the concept of food allergies as they were much less common when they were parents. They may think that allergies are being used as an excuse for failing to manage the not inconsiderable stress of dealing with a newborn, entirely healthy child. It may be helpful to attend clinic appointments with grandparents or other carers to help them with the process of understanding and allow them to ask questions.

> *I think the main impact was worry, from my family, about how I was coping and making sure they could support me however they could. They are now really good at checking ingredients, or checking with me before they give S anything to eat.*

> HANNAH, MUM OF S

> *It makes me angry to think that my son suffered unnecessarily for so long and it breaks my heart when I think about the repercussions that the whole process has had on my husband, Charlie's older sister, Summer, and me. Summer must have sensed something was wrong because, although she was initially excited about having a new baby brother, she started to lash out and become extremely clingy. She began to throw tantrums for the first time and since I was so tired I am ashamed to say that far too often I lost my cool and shouted at my little girl. Everyone was unhappy. I started to resent my husband for not being able to feed our son and lighten the load for me and we would argue constantly. Looking back, I know that my behaviour was symptomatic of the fact that nobody could tell me why my son constantly had a cold and was losing weight and that, although I was to see the GP six more times over the next three months, no one was actually listening to me. My gut instincts were telling me that something was not right with Charlie, that yes, his sister and him were not the same child, but by nine months Charlie was a whole kilogram lighter than his sister was at the same age.*

> THANH, MUM OF CHARLIE

My family, I think, thought I was overreacting. Christmas time with turkey cooked in butter… Surely that'll be ok? – NO! Even today (the boys are coming up to aged four) surely a quarter of a stock cube containing milk in a casserole won't do any harm? – YES, it quite probably will.

EMMA, MUM OF CAMERON AND DILLON

My husband was very reluctant to accept Sam's initial diagnosis and it took a while for it to sink in. Attending the hospital appointments helped a lot.

KATHRYN, MUM OF SAM AND HARRY

Your immediate family must be your priority. Support and full understanding from your partner and an ability to explain to and be there for other children is crucial.

To successfully care for an allergic child, there will be an impact on the whole family. Your immediate family will all have to have some degree of understanding in order to keep your allergic child safe in the home. Whether you change everyone's diets and make family meals that are allergen-free and keep treats and snacks allergen-free, or whether you have separate meals and treats for your allergic child, or whether you do a bit of both, is entirely your choice. Whatever your choice, it will need the support and commitment of your whole family and it needs to be a family decision.

Our other kids have had to change their diets as well. My daughter never knew any different as she is younger. As she has gotten older, she now eats the food Evan is allergic to at school, but is never allowed to bring stuff home.

ERICA, MUM OF EVAN

It is worth remembering that food allergies are rarely not just about the ingestion of food or drink, but can also be about inhalation of cooking food and contact with traces of the allergenic food. You should discuss this sort of contact, and how careful you need to be, with your doctor.

Impact on You

Having a child who is allergic adds to the stress of parenting – an already difficult job – and is bound to take its toll on you.

Coping

It is difficult not to feel like a neurotic, overprotective mother, when actually that is what you are being, because you have to be. I remember the weight of responsibility I felt when I realised that ultimately the only person who would protect Zach every day, was me. At soft play, in someone else's house, at toddler groups, at the library, at singing groups, I had to make sure he didn't lick, eat or touch anything he was allergic or potentially allergic to. It was made even worse by the unknown, not knowing how bad a reaction would be, not knowing the extent of the reaction and exactly what could cause a reaction. Partly I'm fortunate, as I didn't have to share that responsibility. I didn't have to leave Zach with other family members as they live far away, or other carers as I didn't go back to work, so I could ensure he was safe. However, it did affect my trust in other people and I think if I'd have been able to share the load, my anxiety would have been reduced hugely and it would have allowed others to learn how to manage Zach's allergies in the real world, along with me. If it happens again, I will definitely ask for more help.

It is very difficult to share the care of your child with someone else, when the risk of an allergic reaction is so great or so unknown. It is not just about what your child eats, but it is also about the environment she is in, what carers have in their homes, what they are cooking, how clean the toys are that they are playing with and the surfaces they are playing on.

At toddler group, another mum once made a comment to me about how precious I was being about Zach chewing on toys along with the other children, as if I was being over-hygienic. I didn't point out to her that the child who had previously chewed on it had just eaten a biscuit that contained milk and that my child may react badly to that. I just walked away, but two years on, I still remember how judged I felt.

However you cope with the huge changes that are occurring in your life, remember that you are doing your best. You will not know all of the answers or many of the solutions and there will be times when you feel at a complete loss. You will have to learn to trust people, some of whom you have never met before and you will have to learn to strive and keep striving until your child is well, content and thriving. Allow yourself to cry, feel angry and to take a break, but above all, know that it will change, it will improve and you will get there. The next chapter will help you in that process, by talking through ways to manage your child's symptoms and minimise the impact of allergies on your family life.

I shut down as a coping mechanism to get through it. It took me longer to bond properly with the boys. I was a mess, really and couldn't be the mother I wanted to be and the boys needed me to be because there were two of them and I just needed to get them through and keep them well. I was very rigid about routine, how they were looked after and how involved people were. We eventually found a system that kind of worked from an allergy/eczema/asthma point of view and I would not deviate from it for fear of them getting ill again.

EMMA, MUM OF CAMERON AND DILLON

From birth to 12 weeks, I saw three health visitors and four GPs, who all told me that S had colic and told me I was an anxious first-time mum. I feel I was robbed of the first five months of being a mother. I realise these early months are difficult for most mothers, but I felt so isolated especially when we seemed to be surrounded by other babies who seemed so content. I felt that I couldn't comfort my baby and started to panic about being left alone with him, as I feared I couldn't cope. My husband and family were amazing and organised themselves so that I was rarely alone in case S had one of his 'episodes'. I felt overwhelming frustration and disappointment every time I visited a healthcare professional. I was even told by one GP that, as I was a health professional myself, I was looking for problems that weren't there!

HANNAH, MUM OF S

Depression

Depression is a real illness with real symptoms that respond well to the right treatment. It affects different people in different ways and can be caused by a number of things, including life events such as having a baby. Postnatal depression is a specific type of depression linked to having a baby. It is well documented and can be treated. Symptoms of depression include lasting feelings of sadness and hopelessness, losing interest in the things you used to enjoy and feeling very tearful. Often anxiety and depression come together but symptoms can vary.

The health visitor also came to see me as my husband, out of desperation, had called her to say that he thought that I was depressed.

THANH, MUM OF CHARLIE

When our middle son, Finn, was allergic to milk and was very colicky, we found it very hard. All the sleepless nights and crying took its toll on us and in the end we sought support from a counsellor (in fact, we were told by the doctor that it was unlikely anything was wrong and that maybe we should see a counsellor instead!). This time we were more prepared (our first child also had allergies), and because I cut out milk straight away, sleep was better but still not great. We have survived it, although sometimes I wonder if Peter thinks I am mad when I dither 'could these symptoms be because of this… Or that….'.

EMILY, MUM OF FELIX, FINN AND LEO

On my third trip to the GP with Zach, it was suggested that there was nothing wrong with him, but that I was depressed. I knew that I wasn't. There's a vast difference between how I felt because of sleep deprivation, exhaustion, anxiety and fear, because my baby was unwell and clinical depression. The suggestion, however, made me panic even further.

Unfortunately, it can be difficult to distinguish the symptoms of depression from those you may well be feeling anyway as you learn about your baby's symptoms and diagnosis. If any of the feelings mentioned above persist or if any concern you or your partner, it is really important to seek help from your GP.

Exhaustion

During this time with your baby, you will be exhausted and probably more so than other parents with young babies. Support is vital from your partner, extended family and friends, if it is at all available. While really your baby only wants and needs you, as the provider of milk and comfort, try, even for short periods, to have a break and let someone else take over. If you have no other children, or if they are in school, it may also be possible for you to sleep when your baby sleeps in the daytime. Try also to eat well and look after yourself as and when you can. Most importantly, be kind to yourself and try to explain your situation to those around you, even if you don't fully understand it yourself.

> *As the first few weeks went on, Alex was increasingly sick so I took him to the GP and was given Ranitidine. He did seem a little more settled after feeding so I thought we had sussed it, even though he still didn't sleep and still kept being sick. By this point the very lovely health visitor was visiting regularly to support me as I was beyond exhausted. Alex still slept in 20-minute stretches at most and I had a lively and beloved three-year-old who I was trying to give as much attention as she had had before.*
>
> *I used to take them to playgroups smiling but shrugging at the fact that there was always some milky sick on me somewhere. And the smiles didn't seem to go beyond the surface as I mourned the happy, settled baby I had spent many months dreaming of. The medication wasn't working, the screaming was becoming constant and I needed to turn elsewhere for help. Luckily that help DID come in the form of a sensitive and open-minded paediatrician.*
>
> SAM, MUM OF ALEX

Guilt

As a mother, I felt and still do feel that perhaps there are some things that I could have done differently to change things for Zach so that he did not have the allergies that he has. I think it's a natural part of being, not only a parent, but specifically a mother, having carried your child for nine months. Even though I know that there is no evidence to back up my thoughts, I still wonder if something I had done had in some way caused his allergies. I know that it's about genes and therefore there is no blame, but I still do find myself wondering if the choices that I made when I was pregnant, the immunisations that I chose to have during pregnancy or the foods that I craved had any impact on him as he developed. Interestingly, these thoughts don't go and they return with subsequent pregnancies. I am currently eight months pregnant and am full of concern and vigilance about allergy in our unborn child. I do now accept, however, that there is little evidence either way. This has taken some of the responsibility away from me and I have just continued to have a balanced healthy diet and lifestyle.

Self-doubt

I doubted myself hugely. While friends with babies talked about a 'mother's instinct', I felt like I had none. Finally, when the paediatrician referred to Zach as a 'highly distressed little boy whom she was concerned about', all I felt was huge relief. I had been right about Zach, but having a professional say what I had been trying to say for months was almost a vindication. I hadn't been imagining it after all. Self-doubt can have long-lasting effects on how you feel about your role as a parent and how you feel about your ability to meet your child's needs. This may or may not affect your ability to understand and form a bond with your baby. At the back of this book (see page 253) you will find a list of resources that are useful and supportive.

Stress

As for many aspects of parenting, stress and the successful management of that stress is part and parcel of having a child with food allergies. Whether it's the stress of a baby who is distressed, demanding and sleeps poorly, or whether it's the stress of socialising and managing daily events that involve food as your child gets older, food allergies do bring their own challenges to your life as a parent. Successful management of this stress very much depends on your support network and ability to reach out for that support when needed.

Stress was unbelievable. I still don't know how I got through it. Sleep was sporadic – many nights were spent with a red, raw baby cuddling him for comfort, not moving for fear of hurting him and soothing him when he moved as it hurt.

EMMA, MUM OF CAMERON AND DILLON

Since Evan was diagnosed, the biggest impact has been, I would say the stress of keeping the foods away from him at a young age and as he has got older. Also I would say having him in a school environment away from us. I worry all the time when he leaves to go to school. Food is everywhere there. I run my own support group here in Indiana (Michiana Food Allergy & Anaphylaxis Support) but there was not any support here locally. I turned to social media for help. Also, in terms of sleep… what is sleep?

ERICA, MUM OF EVAN

CHAPTER 7
Everyday Allergy Management

The mainstay of allergy management is food avoidance, which must involve education and advice from a registered dietician. When appropriate, your child and child's carers must know how to recognise and treat allergic reactions and there should be an emergency plan in place. The NICE guidelines (2011) recommend that information about which foods to eat and food labelling be given to you before starting an elimination diet. Elimination diets are a great challenge.

As discussed previously, elimination diets, or just living life without allergens, can have social, psychological, financial and nutritional burdens. Food preparation can often be more time-consuming and shopping for allergen-free foods can be more expensive. However, on the positive side, it can also provide a healthier diet for your child and wider family, if carried out correctly and carefully. The dietician again is key in providing both individually tailored education and empowerment to the family and child about ways to live everyday life, while avoiding the food they are allergic to. Living with food allergies is a challenge but can be safe, manageable, nutritional and enjoyable. This chapter runs through the best ways to manage your child's everyday life with food allergies. However, this is no substitute for time spent with an allergy dietician. They may be difficult to get an appointment with but this should not stop you asking.

Become an Expert

•••

Inevitably, you will over time become an expert on what your child can and cannot eat. However, it is worth becoming that expert as early as possible to save time and a lot of stress.

Essentials

- Understand food labels.
- Know the many different names of the allergens that you are looking for.
- Know safe brands, both 'free from' and others.

Know the Names of Allergens and Understand Food Labels

•••

Always check the full ingredients list for allergens and not just the allergy advice box on the food packet. Most, but not all, supermarkets provide 'free from' lists of all of their free from foods. These can often be accessed online from the supermarket's website. Additionally, most supermarkets list ingredients for each food and drink product, as well as allergy information, on their websites. While this can be time-consuming initially, it allows you to order your groceries online or alternatively saves you time when you go to the supermarket. Always check the labels anyway, and make sure that your lists of 'safe' foods and safe brands are up to date (see page 89). Allergy advice boxes are not obligatory on packaging, therefore always read the full ingredients list.

In the European Union, food labelling of 14 allergenic ingredients is compulsory. These regulations, published in 2011, are due to be reviewed and updated in 2014. The new recommendations for labelling will include allergen labelling provision not just for pre-packed foods but also for foods which are sold non-packed or pre-packed for direct sale. The three-year transition period is to allow businesses to make the necessary changes to their processes and labelling designs in order to meet the provisions laid out in the legislation.

The ingredients that require labelling are:

1. **Cereals containing gluten (wheat, rye, barley, oats, spelt and Kamut):** There is no requirement in law for manufacturers to use the term gluten itself in the ingredients list, just the name of the cereal. However, best practice recommends the use of both terms.

2. **Crustaceans (crab, lobster, crayfish, shrimp and prawn):** The common names of the crustaceans are used in labelling.

3. **Egg:** This encompasses all species of eggs, including hen, duck, turkey, quail, goose, gull and guinea fowl.

4. **Fish:** The common fish name will be used in labelling unless there is no common fish species, in which case the generic name 'fish' will be used. A list of common fish names can be found in the Fish Labelling Regulations 2010 (see FSA website, on page 82).

5. **Peanuts:** Includes groundnuts and monkey nuts. Refined and unrefined peanut oil is also labelled with 'peanut'.

6. **Soybeans:** Labelled as 'soya' or 'soy'.

7. **Tree nuts:** Almond, hazelnut, walnut, cashew nut, pecan nut, Brazil nut, pistachio nut, macadamia nut and Queensland nut – the type of nut will be listed in the ingredients panel.

8. **Celery and celeriac:** Refers to any part of the celery plant that has been used.

9. **Mustard:** Refers to the mustard plant and other forms of it.

10. **Sesame seeds:** Includes all products derived from it such as tahini and houmous.

11. **Sulphites (in concentrations over 10 parts per million):** Labelling is only required if it has been deliberately added in the preparation of the food. Referred to as 'sulphur dioxide' or 'sulphites'. The chemical name may also be used.

12. **Milk (including lactose):** Dairy products such as cheese, butter, yoghurt and cream may not have milk labelled. However, milk needs to be clearly labelled in unfamiliar dairy products such as mascarpone or fromage frais, and in products in non-transparent packaging where the name does not clearly refer to milk. Components of milk such as casein or whey should be declared with reference to milk.

13. **Lupin:** There is cross-reactivity to lupin in a significant number of people allergic to peanuts. The term is used for both lupin seed and lupin flour.

14. **Molluscs (oysters, clams, mussels, squid, abalone, octopus and snail):** The name of the mollusc is used in labelling unless it is a rare mollusc, in which case the generic term 'mollusc' will be used. For common molluscs please see the Fish Labelling Regulations 2010 (see FSA website, below).

The Food Standards Agency (FSA), in its guidance to food manufacturers, producers, retailers and caterers, recommends that the common names for allergens are used in labelling. The definitive source to food labelling can be found on the FSA website http://food.gov.uk/policy-advice/allergyintol/

Advisory Warning Labels (AWLs)

Many manufacturers provide advice about the potential for unintentional contamination with allergens. However, the absence of a 'may contain', also known as an advisory warning label (AWL), does not indicate that a food is free of potential cross-contaminants. The use of AWLs on packaged foods is voluntary. This means that there are huge inconsistencies in labelling between manufacturers, within product categories and between different countries.

While awareness of the dangers posed by allergenic foods has increased within the food industry over the past 20 years, understanding is still far from complete. Foods can become contaminated with residues of allergenic foods at many points along the food chain, including harvesting on farms, storage, transportation and during manufacture. Typically, different products may be produced on the same equipment line, some containing allergenic products and others not. While many companies make efforts to clean shared equipment between product runs, this is not the case for all manufacturers and the effectiveness of such approaches is unclear.

There are reports in the medical literature (see References pages 281) of potentially life-threatening reactions due to peanut contamination in confectionery and biscuit products without AWLs. On the basis of this, it is assumed that the presence of an advisory warning does not indicate the contamination risk, or, the absence of an advisory warning label is not indicative of no or even low risk of contamination.

In the Resources chapter at the back of this book (see pages 271–79) is a table of the major food allergens and other names to also look out for when reading food labels and ingredients. It is worth signing up to the allergen alert services, such as those by the FSA at http://food.gov.uk/policy-advice/allergyintol/alerts/#.UkQANBZTE20 or the Anaphylaxis Campaign (http://www.anaphylaxis.org.uk/living-with-anaphylaxis/product-alerts) for product safety alerts.

Risk levels

Remember that every allergic child is different, not just in exactly what they need to avoid but also the degree of avoidance required. Children with non-IgE mediated reactions (see page 5) are not at risk of anaphylaxis (see page 6) and when symptoms are mild, you may even choose to introduce small amounts of the food into their diet and manage symptoms such as eczema with steroid creams. However, this is in stark contrast to the child with multiple IgE type food allergies (see page 4) and a history of severe reactions with asthma, who has a high risk of anaphylaxis and needs to have far more stringent avoidance strategies. Even among children with immediate allergies, there is a difference in levels of risk. For example, a child with egg or milk allergy who is already able to tolerate the foods in the baked form may be at lower risk of severe reactions. You may be able to adopt a different approach to allergen avoidance, especially in foods carrying advisory labels.

Two things are important when considering avoidance. Firstly, discuss the issue of allergen avoidance, specific to your situation and your child, with your specialist and dietician. Secondly, develop the skills of risk assessment.

Risk assessment

As a parent you need clear labelling of food products with possible allergen contamination so that you can make an informed decision about the level of risk that you may take. However, clear labelling is not available. It is not even the case that the wording on the AWL gives useful information as to the potential for cross-contamination in a product. A label that says 'may contain' and a label that says 'made in a factory that uses…' are no different in the information that they provide and therefore they hold no weight in terms of risk assessment for the potential of cross-contamination of the allergen in that food. The ability of your child therefore to tolerate foods that have an AWL should not be interpreted as reflecting a mild nature of their allergy and thinking as such could put them at risk of a severe allergic reaction. Tolerating a food with an AWL is most likely because none of the allergen found its way into the product. The risk assessment that you make as a parent relies not just on the likelihood of contamination, but also whether the degree of contamination is sufficient to provoke an allergic reaction in your child.

Health professionals also need to take into consideration a host of factors when making a risk assessment in order to provide you with appropriate advice with regards to AWLs. The most important factor is considering your child's allergies individually. For each child, the balance between nutritional requirements, quality of life and risk needs to be carefully assessed. Specialist paediatric dietetic input is crucial for your child and family. In addition to ensuring that your child has a nutritionally adequate diet, specialist dietetic advice linked specifically to your child's allergies, along with the advice and support available through an allergy clinic, will allow you to be better informed and therefore can reduce the risk to your child of an accidental reaction.

The majority of fatal allergic reactions to peanuts occur outside the home environment and, on this basis, additional caution is recommended when eating unfamiliar foods in an unfamiliar environment, irrespective of the presence or absence of AWLs. It may be best for your child to follow more stringent dietary avoidance when outside the home environment. The extent to which a health professional might recommend avoidance of products with AWLs should depend on a range of factors, including the presence or absence of risk factors for severe reactions and the availability of and familiarity with emergency rescue medication.

As the parent trying to shop for your child, labelling has big implications and it may be one of the reasons why you choose to prepare and cook at home. Due to the ongoing risks of exposure, it is important to recognise the early symptoms of an allergic reaction and treat it appropriately. Reactions will happen from time to time, it is almost inevitable. It doesn't mean that you have failed, but it is important to try to learn lessons. Thankfully, severe reactions are rare.

Education should extend to members of the community, such as teachers and school nurses. You and your child should receive information about patient support groups, which often have useful online resources. In order to be able to treat anaphylaxis in the community, your child needs to be prescribed an adrenaline autoinjector. This and all the issues above need to be discussed with your doctor.

Be Prepared and Don't Panic

All parents prepare, perhaps that's one of the main tasks of managing a child's day, but for your allergic child preparation is vital and becomes the key to staying safe. Cross-contamination, where allergens are transferred to otherwise non-allergenic areas in the home, is a risk with food allergies. Here are some ways to manage this risk.

- If prescribed, ensure your two adrenaline autoinjectors (known as AAIs) are always easily accessible and in date.
- Always have antihistamine available, perhaps one bottle upstairs and one downstairs.
- Prepare allergy-free food first before preparing other food.
- Use separate chopping boards, cheese graters, knives, etc. for food preparation.
- Teach your children to wash their hands before and after eating, along with the rest of the family.

- Use a separate shelf in your fridge for allergy-free food, preferably on the top shelf.

- Try to make allergy-free recipes for the whole family (see Chapter 16 for lots of recipe ideas).

- Store foods separately to prevent cross-contamination.

- Keep open allergenic foods in closed containers.

- Keep allergy-free sweet treats in a separate container.

- Use a hot dishwasher cycle to clean all utensils.

- If washing by hand, wash your allergic child's plates and cutlery before others in hot, soapy water.

- Check your washing-up liquid ingredients – we found that ours contained whey.

- Use clean kitchen roll to wipe surfaces, not the same dishcloth as you use to clean other surfaces.

- Clean spills with warm, soapy water or an antibacterial spray.

- Clean the table and under the table.

- Be cautious when cooking allergenic foods as your child could react. Some families completely exclude the allergen from the home environment to reduce risk but this obviously impacts on the rest of the family. Discuss whether this is necessary with your doctor.

- Check ingredients on all products, not just food. Cosmetics, medication, handwash, as well as pet food, can all contain allergens.

- Be aware of high-risk cross-contamination situations such as barbeques, deli counters, self-service salad bars and pre-packaged sandwiches.

Be organised

It is difficult to be prepared and organised when you are anxious and sleep deprived. However, a few bits of organisation, like writing notes to remember your questions for healthcare professionals and preparing shopping lists and writing down ingredients, can help enormously in the daily management of your child's allergies.

> *If I could rewind and start again, I would have written everything down so when I went to the healthcare advisors, the GP and the allergy test I would have felt more in control and not got so flustered. If I had the phone call from the dietician again, I would ask her to put her advice in writing and taken it to the allergy test with me.*
>
> EMMA, MUM OF HUNTER

Whatever the circumstances, whether it is preparing your child for nursery and preparing the nursery for your allergic child, managing trips to friends or family, to a restaurant or party, planning and preparation are key. Once you accept that, it quickly becomes second nature.

> *Always read labels and make sure your children or child always has his or her medication. Start that at a young age. My son has self-carried since he turned five years old. Ask many questions when at doctor visits, even take notes if you have to. Remind doctors and hospital staff of your child's allergens as they can be overlooked. Be consistent with holidays and meals, always. Never let your guard down. Never stop educating people. Be firm, but not rude (it can be hard). Help your school. Schools are for the most part clueless. They need guidance to help. Try to remember that you have taught your child well. It's hard to let go. My oldest is 21 and it was hard to let him go even without food allergies. Trust that children will do what*

you have taught them, even if it is reminding them daily to carry their medication.

ERICA, MUM OF EVAN

Meal plan

As all organised and busy parents will tell you, a meal plan is a must! With your allergic child, it is even more of a must. Try to plan a week ahead if you can. That way you can seek to ensure your child gets a nutritionally varied diet over the week, at least within the limited range of safe foods.

Food shopping

The safest way to shop is to buy fresh, unprocessed food. However, we all use processed food at some point! Make a list of safe food for each meal and safe snacks. Keep the list somewhere handy so that you can add to it as you go through the weaning process. Not only is it a helpful reminder and prompt for you when shopping and meal planning, but it is also encouraging as you can see the list of safe foods growing. Hand the list out to family or friends. Remember to specify food brands, as different brands contain different ingredients. For example, Heinz Tomato Ketchup has no dairy, Co-operative own brand does. Remarkably, even different-sized packets of the same food may have different ingredients and ingredients also change for the same product so you need to stay alert.

Know Safe Brands

The 'free from' food market is expanding all the time. Some brands cater for specific allergies and others for a wide range, producing food that not only removes all major allergens, but is tasty as well. These brands are sold by specialist retailers as well as in major supermarkets. It is very helpful to get to know these brands as well as their stockists (see Resources pages 256–8). Even with 'free from' foods, always read the label to find out which allergens have been removed.

Commercial baby foods

Even though your baby or toddler has allergies, he can still eat some commercially available baby foods. Many brands have allergen-free varieties, which can make life a bit easier. They are all clearly labelled and generally nutritious. They include purées, juices, smoothies, snacks and toddler meals. They can therefore be used throughout weaning and as your child gets older.

Whether you are a home cook or not, it is always nice to have an alternative solution to make life less busy. You could also use these bought baby foods as the basis of a meal and add your own fresh ingredients to increase flavour, texture and nutritional content.

Note: Manufacturers do change food ingredients. Therefore, never assume that the ingredients are the same. *Every time you buy a product, read the label.*

'Free from' food brands

'Free from' food brands are on the increase. There is a list of some of them and which foods they produce in the Resources chapter at the back of this book (see pages 256–8). It is worth remembering, however, that many foods not in the 'free from' section may also be suitable for your child.

Allergies have changed our lives. We check food labels and have to be so careful... We pack food whenever we go out so that if the kids get hungry we have something to feed them. There is no shop that we can go to and get 'fast food' for my son.

ANNE, MUM OF HANNAH AND EDWARD

The Wider World

For the majority of the parents that I spoke to in preparing this book, the biggest fear was leaving their child. However, separation from the parent and inclusion in wider social networks are both vital parts of the process of childhood. To be secure even when separated for a while is part of growing up. However, the additional angst of allergies and anaphylaxis looms over any sense of peaceful, happy and independent activity for the parent and possibly for the child. A careful and timely balance between separation and anxiety has to be found.

My biggest worry is leaving him on his own in the care of his school once I am no longer there. Currently I stay in the building and help at the school but in a couple of years that will no longer happen and that terrifies me. I am worried people will not act quickly enough when it is needed.

BEV, MUM OF LEVI

In short, any situation with food involved outside of the home and outside of my immediate family is anxiety provoking for me, I just hope I have hidden it well enough from the boys that they are not anxious.

EMMA, MUM OF CAMERON AND DILLON

Below are some tried-and-tested ideas to make this process as safe and fearless as possible. These precautions are mainly indicated if your child has immediate, IgE mediated allergies.

1. Your bag essentials

Medication: Never leave home without your child's medication. I carry an antihistamine and the adrenaline autoinjector with me at all times, together with our written emergency plan (which has been laminated). I never remove it and always take the same bag with me so I know where it is at all times. Involve your child in this process from an early age, so he too can take some responsibility for it.

> *From the beginning, teach your child never to leave home without prescribed medications. Being prepared for an allergic reaction is the key to a safe life.*
>
> THE ANAPHYLAXIS CAMPAIGN, 2008

Antibacterial wipes: Always pack some sterile wipes to clean surfaces that may be contaminated.

Allergen-free sweet treats: Keep these to hand to give to your child if friends are having a treat too. This way there is no sense of being left out.

2. Written emergency plan

Any child with a diagnosed food allergy should have a formal emergency treatment plan in place. The British Society for Allergy and Clinical Immunology has produced standard UK plans which are available for healthcare professionals on their website www.bsaci.org

A written, personal emergency plan should be provided for a childminder, nursery preschool or school. There is an example in the Resources chapter at the end of this book (see pages 260–4).

3. Register your adrenaline autoinjector

When you receive your EpiPen or Jext autoinjector, the number and expiry date can be registered. You will then receive email and or text alerts giving one month, then weekly notifications that the autoinjector is about to expire, giving plenty of time to get a replacement. See www.EpiPen.com and www.jext.co.uk for more information.

4. Medical identification

For younger children wristbands from Mediband are brilliant, they look cool and they are a constant visual reminder to friends, family and carers.

MEL, MUM OF E

Alert bracelets don't have to single out your child but can work as a prompt for the caregiver and provide you with some peace of mind. There are some great designs available for children. See the Resources chapter at the back of this book (see page 258) for more information.

5. Educate your family and friends

Your child has food allergies and although it is important to create a safe environment for them to be in, it is also vital to teach your child from an early age about their allergies. The dilemma for parents is at what age is it best to do this and how should it be done? How much detail should you go into? How do you empower and inform your child without frightening him? How do you tell him that what he eats is different without making him *feel* different? Above all, how do you keep your own fears at bay and just teach your child the facts?

Family are supportive now – it is 'official'– as are friends but before we had seen the consultant sometimes I got the impression that maybe I was making life difficult for myself?! Also as the symptoms weren't obvious anaphylactic ones it maybe was harder for people to grasp. I did have meals at friends' houses and having told them I couldn't eat dairy because of Felix still found myself with food that had cheese or cream in it (that isn't dairy is it??!!). It is easier now it is just Felix, because people always ask before they offer a toddler food – or at least have done so far! Felix's brothers think it is funny that Felix has one type of 'milk', Finn another and Leo yet another but I think that also makes them feel a bit special.

EMILY, MUM OF FELIX, FINN AND LEO

We have struggled a little with parents/older generation taking it seriously and getting their heads around what they can and can't eat. Even now, four years on, we are still given products containing nuts at Christmas. Some others have thought we are making a fuss or even making it up. I have had to go through the whole story with one person who thought it was all in my head. It surprises me that people don't understand that these are potentially life-threatening conditions.

KATHRYN, MUM OF SAM AND HARRY

Evan has yet to go to a birthday party without us. When he does go, we take his own food. On holiday, I always bring food for him as it's hard to accommodate when others don't 'get it'. My house is completely allergy-free for him. We do go out to eat occasionally, but always call ahead or go where we know it is safe. I have been known to go into a kitchen at a restaurant and read labels! As he has got older, he tends not to want to eat out.

ERICA, MUM OF EVAN

It is entirely up to you if you want to make your home environment allergy-free or whether you just have separate foods for your allergic child. Some parents that I spoke to make the home allergy-free in order to allow their child complete freedom in the home and freedom from worry for them as parents. Others don't do this and use the home environment as a mirror for the outside world, where your child will come into contact with allergens. There are advantages to both ways, but whatever you decide, education is still the way forward.

Allergies scare my parents, but they are getting more confident with time and as my son gets older he is easier to deal with and he has an amazing sixth sense of what will hurt him and make him sick.

ANNE, MUM OF HANNAH AND EDWARD

Friends and family are sympathetic, but scared. Everyone worries about an anaphylactic reaction and they check everything with me.

MEL, MUM OF E

We tend to not leave the children with anyone besides our family. People were terrible and some still are. We get the 'Oh it's just hives, give him some Benadryl'. Or 'Just give him a little bit to build up his immune system'. Our wider family has learned over the years to accept it, but sometimes still does not understand it. People at school still think I am crazy and overreact... Some people choose to understand and others don't.

ERICA, MUM OF EVAN

Although it is difficult, there are some benefits to allowing other members of the family to eat a 'normal' diet. It is a fact of life that your allergic child has to grow up knowing that other people eat different things and that there are some things they themselves cannot eat. It is a reality for your allergic child, so preparing him in the home for life outside is essential. Family members can learn how to safely eat food and clean up afterwards without excluding the allergic child.

> *It has been a hard journey but we have two lovely kids and my daughter is very aware of her allergies and asks what is in food. My husband has been very supportive; it would have been a much harder journey without him. My parents have been very supportive. Other family members don't seem to get it and don't understand the consequences of getting it wrong if the kids have something they are allergic to. I guess we visit those family members but don't stay long.*

ANNE, MUM OF HANNAH AND EDWARD

6. Educate your child

As parents, we are responsible for preparing our children for life outside the home. The list is endless – learning social skills, how to play together, take turns, be patient and for your allergic child learning about safe and unsafe foods, treatments that work and the names of allergens is part of that preparation. Teach your child to know what he can and cannot eat and to ask for help if he does not know. Even from an early age, you can teach your child to ask if the food contains an allergen. This will empower your child, allowing him to feel in control and it will help to relieve your anxiety as a parent. It is important that your child feels in control, involved and part of the treatment regimes and food avoidance that he is following. Talking and playing are good ways to help your child learn and can help to reduce anxiety for both you and your child.

It is unrealistic to expect that one day we will sit down with our children and pass on the control of their allergies. The fact is that letting go and teaching responsibility is a process that will develop over years... It is important to start teaching children as soon as possible about avoiding certain foods, and knowing what to do if they eat something they react to.

Whatever works for you, remember that the goal is to provide your child with a sense of control over the allergy, and to realise that he or she has options... Be careful of the language you use when you talk about the dangers. Although it's important to convey seriousness, constant references to death will not help.

THE ANAPHYLAXIS CAMPAIGN, 2008

Inevitably there will be times when your child's quality of life suffers due to poor sleep, difficulty breathing, sore skin and so on. However, if your child feels confident about his allergies and understands the treatments that can help him, with encouragement, his feelings about his condition can be discussed, acknowledged and talked about positively.

Zach loves Thomas the Tank Engine and we recently saw an episode where Henry, one of the engines, gets sick, red in the face and starts to puff and wheeze. No one knows why he is sick until he says it's because he had the wrong coal! It was a useful way for me to talk about eggs and dairy and how despite being allergic to coal, Henry was still a really useful engine. Zach smiled and asked to watch the episode again and again... six times in all!

There are great websites and books for different-aged children that can help in explaining and talking to your child. I have included some of them in the Resources chapter at the back of this book (see page 256).

Cooking and eating with your child is a great way to educate him as well. I once heard a play therapist say that children talk best while doing something, and cooking is ideal. Rather than pointing out what your child *cannot* eat, have specific times when you cook and eat food that your child *can* eat. It then becomes a positive difference. Children learn that they have soya milk not cow's milk and they learn to recognise cartons and labels before they can even read. They can learn what eggs look like but that they don't cook or eat them in cakes, for example. If you start this gentle, informal process early then differences in the foods that people can and cannot eat becomes a natural, normal part of life, not an emphasised negative part.

> *He's a good boy really, takes it all in his stride and mummy bakes him treats every now and then so he doesn't feel left out. One day soon he will start to realise he is a little different from the other kids at school but for now I don't think he realises, and hopefully we can work around those future issues the best way possible so he feels happy with it all.*

BEV, MUM OF LEVI

7. Educate the nursery, preschool and school

Schools and many preschools and nurseries will have training procedures and protocols in place for the management of other children's food and for the management of a child with food allergies and anaphylaxis. Get hold of a copy of these, read and ask any questions that you have. If your child's school has concerns about managing your child's allergies, please see the Anaphylaxis Campaign for key recommendations made for schools in 2010 (http://www.anaphylaxis.org.uk/schools/help-for-schools).

My biggest fear now is that Hunter will have a reaction while at nursery, despite filling in detailed forms and discussing it with his key worker. I can't quite trust that they will ensure the food is safe. As a result Hunter has not stayed at nursery for lunch to date, but this is something I know I need to deal with eventually.

EMMA, MUM OF HUNTER

My son has been in childcare since he was six months old. His carers have been amazing. The first time we took him in for a settling visit, the carer cuddled him and put him in a cot for a sleep. He reacted to the laundry powders and got a red rash on his cheeks and exposed skin that touched the clothes and cot... He did have a couple of food reactions in those initial periods but mainly to skin contact and that is still the case. He stayed in the babies' room for one-and-a-half years and eventually moved up when he got an EpiPen autoinjector...

ANNE, MUM OF HANNAH AND EDWARD

Before your child starts nursery, preschool or school, arrange to visit in person and ideally meet with your child's class teacher as well as the headteacher and other key members of staff. Talk to the staff about your child's allergies and about the precautions that have to be taken. It is also important to provide a written emergency plan, clearly stating the foods that your child cannot have and going through the emergency procedure step by step. It is useful to include a photo of your child on this form. There is an example written plan for preschool in the Resources chapter at the back of this book (see page 261).

As the parent, you will need to provide the appropriate medication for your child, which should always have your child's name on the pharmacy label. It is useful to keep this all together in a named container for ease and safety of storage. You are responsible for making sure this medication has not passed its expiry date and replacing it, if necessary. Try to ensure that as many staff are aware of it as possible and that there are identified AAI administrator trained staff always available. The most important staff members to educate are your child's class teacher and teaching assistant, those involved with your child every day. Do all you can to revisit when, where and how to use the AAI at regular intervals. Medicines can only be given with prior written consent of the parents. Provide your child's written emergency plan (see pages 47–8). When the medicine is required, the staff must feel able to act in the place of you the parent and should have no fear or ambiguity about giving the medicine when needed. The medicine to manage an allergic reaction will not harm your child if given when not strictly necessary. What will harm your child is not giving it when it is needed.

Often a healthcare professional can help facilitate the process of teaching the school about anaphylaxis and allergy management. Speak to your health visitor, GP or allergist for further help.

With nursery you need to have a meeting with them before your child starts. Make posters with YES and NO foods. Make it as easy for them as possible. Provide strict and specific instructions for which reactions require which medicine and actions etc.

BEV, MUM OF LEVI

There are training DVDs available and websites that provide specific school and preschool age-appropriate teaching material. There are online training courses called AllergyWise designed for individuals, carers, families, employers and healthcare professionals. There are also specifically designed courses for healthcare professionals, including GPs, practice nurses and pharmacists that are run by the Anaphylaxis Campaign (www.anaphylaxis.org.uk).

Most importantly, teach your child about which member of staff to go to if he is feeling unwell.

Food

Younger children who are unable to read food labels should be taught not to share food. Risk assessment is a skill that needs to be learned early in life. Rather than ban certain foods, it may be of more value for schools to encourage children to be aware of what they eat, what their friends can and cannot eat and to recognise signs of an allergic reaction.

Education can help reduce anxiety and fear and instil confidence in the ability to cope in the event of anaphylaxis.

Zach was due to start preschool in the September, so the preschool and I arranged a training session for all the staff, run by the allergy and asthma clinical nurse specialist from the local hospital. All the staff attended, along with a community paediatric nurse from the GP surgery. The topics discussed were allergy, anaphylaxis and practice at using the EpiPen. My husband and I were able to talk about Zach and the foods to avoid and how we manage every day. The staff then did a problem-solving session where they discussed solutions for snack time, birthdays, baking and junk modelling (see page 102). The aim of the session was inclusion of Zach and as a family we went away feeling supported and positive. Everyone was willing to help and I didn't feel like a nuisance at all. As a result they changed their birthday cake policy and used allergy-free baking recipes. Zach sits at the water end of the table during snack time and puts his plate and cup on top of the trolley when he has finished, rather than in the washing-up bowl along with the other children.

Snack time

Discuss where your child will sit during snack time and what snacks are available. Provide separate snacks for your child, if necessary. If milk will be available, where will your child sit and where will he put his plate and cup at the end? Could there be designated water and milk ends of the table so that your child sits at the water end? How will spills be dealt with?

Baking

Provide replacements for baking and offer to help if at all possible.

Junk modelling

Does the school use old egg, milk, flour and chocolate boxes and cartons for crafts? If so, can alternatives be used when your child is there?

Parties and Social Events

I tend to run through an emergency plan in my head when going out or planning to leave Zach with grandparents. I will always go through the use of the autoinjector with others and clearly state that an ambulance will need to be called. If Zach is going to a children's party, I always speak to someone else such as a relative or friend if my husband isn't there to help me if there is a crisis. It's good to have a back-up and someone who will call an ambulance or care for other children should the need arise. I never leave Zach unsupervised at parties.

Children's parties are a minefield of emotions. As a parent, you want your child to be included and not feel different to anyone else, but the reality is that he is different. It is very unlikely that your child will be able to eat the birthday cake or the chocolates and biscuits, sandwiches, dips and snacks on offer. However, the good news is that with some careful planning and distraction, a child will notice a difference but not significantly so. The difference will hopefully not make him sad and that surely is what we as parents really hope for.

Children seem to be excellent at accepting. If your child understands that a certain food will make him poorly, he is likely to be happy to accept a cake or chocolate substitute. Try to speak to the host beforehand if you can and come prepared with an array of substitutes if at all possible.

Birthday parties are often avoided unless I know the parents (again fear of looking like a neurotic mother). I make chocolate cupcakes for the boys so they don't miss out on cake and check what is going to be available and take party type food for them if needed. The most scary birthday party situation was at my nephew's third birthday party – there was a piñata filled with chocolate and sweets that the boys couldn't have. My sister did have chocolate for the boys so they could still eat some. But a floor covered in chocolate and children covered in chocolate was scary for me and I really struggled with whether to let the boys join in picking up the chocolate coins or not! My sister is wonderful and always has food for the boys and has more [safe] chocolate for them in her house than I have in my house!

EMMA, MUM OF CAMERON AND DILLON

My daughter goes to birthday parties, which I find challenging. We take her own cake and call ahead to ensure that the host is aware of Hannah's allergies. I stay and make sure that she does not eat anything that will cause a reaction as little macaroons are often served – these can make her very sick.

ANNE, MUM OF HANNAH AND EDWARD

Party survival tips

- Contact the host before the party, if possible, and ask what food will be provided. That way you can take similar alternatives with you.

- Accept help. If the host offers to provide for your child, give a list of safe foods or try to provide similar snacks for your child so that they can be included.

- Have an ally. Ask a friend to help you keep an eye on your child.

- Check party bags for sweets, biscuits and chocolates and try to replace them with allergy-friendly alternatives.

- Go prepared – party games often include chocolates and sweets. Take alternatives for your child.

- Accept that you have to be extra vigilant. You are not being an overprotective parent. You are being responsible for your child's safety.

- Run through a 'what if...' plan in your head or with a friend/partner/relative for the worst-case scenario.

- Don't allow your child to share cups, drinking straws and utensils with other children.

- If another child uses your child's things, discreetly remove it or clean with a sterile surface wipe.

- Keep a few cupcakes in the freezer, so you are prepared. Defrost, decorate and take a cupcake with you to the party, just for your child.

- Allow yourself to do whatever you need to to ensure your child's safety.

I tend to take a 'special treat' if we are somewhere where other children have cake or biscuits so that S feels he is also having something different and exciting. I found a dairy- and egg-free cake recipe online for his first birthday cake as it was very important to me that he should have a cake. I thought I would use this recipe to make little cakes to take to future parties so that he isn't left out.

HANNAH, MUM OF S

Toddler Groups/Soft Play

Use antibacterial wipes on any toys or surfaces that your child may come into contact with. Take biscuits and drinks with you to cater for snack time the first time that you go. On subsequent visits, ask about the brand of biscuits used at snack time and then check the labels of those brands in the supermarket. The aim is to allow your child to be as included as possible. Occasionally, the provided snack may be a safe option.

Eating Out

In a restaurant, the risk of cross-contamination is great and so you may want to have a discussion with the chef or waiting staff. But some restaurants, especially chain ones, can be very allergy-wise. Some provide their own ingredients lists that are allergy specific for each meal. You can find these online or by asking the waiter or better still the chef or manager. It can be useful to phone ahead to discuss provision for your child. It may be a good idea to use a 'chef card', such as those available from www.dietarycard.co.uk. Hand the card to your waiter to pass on to the chef. Most restaurants are very accommodating. If in doubt, always take your child's meal with you as well as your own snacks.

When eating out we take a plate of food made up as close as possible to what the rest of us will have – for example, pizza for a pizza restaurant.

BEV, MUM OF LEVI

We do enjoy eating out and have generally found restaurants to be very helpful. What doesn't help is the constant use of 'we can't guarantee' etc. One waiter at a Jamie Oliver restaurant was great, he sat down with us and explained all the risks, what was used and the areas of potential cross-contamination.

KATHRYN, MUM OF SAM AND HARRY

Meals out are rare as it is so difficult and unpredictable in terms of whether the boys can eat and I am fearful of arriving somewhere with two hungry toddlers and no food! Also I do struggle with trusting waiting/bar staff to relay messages and the chef to be careful of cross-contamination. So many people hear 'intolerance' when I say 'allergy'. My best friend is good at saying, 'You do have their EpiPens with you, don't you?' when we order food – that normally gets the gravity of a reaction across quite nicely.

EMMA, MUM OF CAMERON AND DILLON

Top tips for eating out

- Carry an allergy-safe chocolate treat around with you, so that you can always join in with the spontaneous sweet treat or provide your child with a much-loved dessert option.

- Carry an allergy-free tomato ketchup sachet with you. Unlabelled brands often contain milk protein.
- In addition to medication, carry antibacterial wipes with you for cleaning surfaces, such as highchairs and tables, which may come into contact with your child's skin.

Note of caution: Certain styles of eating such as buffet and salad bars have an increased risk of cross-contamination. Asian and other ethnic restaurants tend to use more allergenic ingredients such as nuts and sesame seeds.

Travel

With a little careful planning, it is possible to travel safely with an allergic child. Translation cards are available and are well worth buying if you are going abroad with your child. These wallet-sized cards are available from Allergy UK in a range of languages. The cards specify the foods that your child is allergic to. They are therefore great when eating out. There is also an emergency card if your child is having an anaphylactic reaction. It says what is happening to your child and that you need an ambulance.

Holidays have been more challenging, especially in places which use a lot of dairy. We have just had to be very organised about preparing his food and self-cater where possible.

HANNAH, MUM OF S

We have taken Sam to France. We self-catered and ate out. My husband's French is pretty good and he made sure he asked every time what the food contained and stated that it was a severe allergy. We haven't yet taken Harry abroad – we are considering it but the milk allergy is so much harder.

KATHRYN, MUM OF SAM AND HARRY

Make sure that you have enough of your child's medication to take with you on holiday. If travelling abroad, your child's medication must be carried on the plane and kept with you at all times in the hand luggage. Liquid restrictions at airports and the airlines themselves will require that you carry a letter from your GP or allergist stating your child's name, allergies and reasons for carrying the specified medication. Often GPs charge for this service, so it is worth getting the wording right the first time. Please see the Resources section (see page 264) for a travel letter example. Contact your airport or airline for further details and also to see if a suitable meal can be provided for your child. Take snacks with you in case of delay but avoid meat and be aware that only small amounts of fruit or vegetables are allowed abroad.

Before you reach your destination, find out about the emergency services in the country and the nearest hospital. For shopping, be aware that food-labelling rules vary outside the EU. It is useful to keep the translated names of your child's allergenic foods with you for supermarket shopping.

We went to France for my sister's wedding in January 2010. I took long-life soya milk, soya custard and some soya puddings with me. My sister very kindly put us in an apartment so I could cook for the boys while everyone else was in the hotel. I bought fresh food (fruit, veg and meat) and cooked for them and learned how to check about allergy-inducing food in French so that we could buy bread.

EMMA, MUM OF CAMERON AND DILLON

Separation and Independence

Anxiety about your child's safety can be huge when your child suffers from allergies because normal activities can pose huge dangers. However, separation and independence are a natural, vital part of growing up. It is important to talk to those you trust about your fears and anxieties.

I feel nervous about leaving Levi with people, so generally if he wants to go to a friend's or to a party I go along too. It is very hard to trust others with the amount of responsibility and things to remember. I think it is true to say that it can cause separation anxiety for the mother as well as the allergic child. I do trust my partner, however, and I know that if he is unsure he will always ask first.

BEV, MUM OF LEVI

The biggest impact was, and still is, the fear that the boys will have a life-threatening reaction – going to play group/soft play/the park, where other children are eating and might drop something. I fear they will be given something, or pick up something to eat that will cause a reaction. Birthday parties are a minefield and I feel like a neurotic mother! It is hard to let them go and explore the world with such potential for harm. What if they are in the middle of soft play and have a reaction and I'm not with them?! What if someone is looking after them and they forget to take the EpiPens out?! What if we are eating away from home and there is cross-contamination in the kitchen because people aren't as careful as I am?!

EMMA, MUM OF CAMERON AND DILLON

I suppose the biggest impact is that we rarely leave them both. I have never used a childminder. There are a handful of very close people we can trust to look after them. We are entering a new era of school with Sam, which is quite stressful and we worry that he is singled out as different to his classmates.

KATHRYN, MUM OF SAM AND HARRY

As previously discussed, try to empower your child by teaching them, playing games with them that involve pretend food allergens and scenarios that they might come up against when they are without you, so that they have practised how to respond and feel confident. Try to make the environment around them as safe as possible by educating those around them and remember to praise your child for learning about and coping with their symptoms. Your child may inevitably pick up on your anxieties but it is important that he has the self-esteem and confidence to enjoy and live his life. As a parent, all you can do is your best and allergies are like any other difficulty your child may face in life and as such can be tackled and overcome positively.

Modify your strategies, as your child grows older. Keeping things too simple may hinder your child's ownership of the allergy but if your expectations are set above the child's capability, your child may feel defeated. Overprotection can send the signal that you think your child is not capable of handling situations. You will need to search for a balance that's right for your family.

THE ANAPHYLAXIS CAMPAIGN, 2008

CHAPTER 8
Anaphylactic Reaction

Anaphylaxis is defined as a serious allergic reaction that is rapid in onset and may cause death. It is the most extreme form of an IgE mediated reaction (see page 4). The incidence of anaphylaxis is rare but seems to be increasing. Parents and healthcare professionals, such as paramedics, need to be familiar with anaphylaxis to ensure that management is the best that it can be. The most effective treatment of anaphylaxis is the prompt administration of adrenaline using an autoinjector (see page 118).

Recognising what is happening to your child early on is key. Once the reaction is over, appropriate follow-up with thorough investigation into the cause, if unknown, and advice on future prevention is also crucial. As the parent, you and your child can be empowered to understand what is triggering your child's reactions and learn about the day-to-day role of effectively managing anaphylaxis.

> *Levi's nut and egg allergies have shown the most severe reaction so far with wheezing and swelling. He carries an EpiPen for these.*
>
> BEV, MUM OF LEVI

In children, the most common cause of anaphylaxis is food allergy and the most common symptoms are severe breathing difficulties. In adults, reactions to drugs such as antibiotics, latex or insect stings are more common causes. These reactions are all very rare in children. It is not possible to predict who may suffer an anaphylactic reaction, as the severity of the allergic reaction is dependent on lots of factors. Allergic reactions to food are unpredictable and anyone with an IgE mediated food allergy (see page 4), in the wrong set of circumstances, may have a severe reaction. Previous severe reactions are a risk factor for future anaphylaxis but there is no evidence that allergic reactions become progressively more severe with subsequent exposures to the allergen – despite the myth about this. If your child has other illnesses, especially asthma, there is a link with a more severe allergic reaction to food allergens.

To recognise a food-allergic reaction in your child and to respond with appropriate treatments, it is important to know and consider both the symptoms of an allergic reaction that are not harmful, although they may be uncomfortable, as well as the symptoms that are already, or may soon become, life-threatening.

An Allergic Reaction

The stories below are not anaphylaxis but they are allergic reactions. It is important to be clear about the difference.

> *Hannah's first reaction occurred just before Christmas. We had made a cake containing walnuts and she ate a tiny amount and went out to the garden. After about 35–40 minutes I noticed she was scratching… I took her inside and rang the 24-hour nurse. They said take her to hospital and call an ambulance if her reaction got worse. We jumped in the car and took her to hospital and then the triage nurse examined her and gave her some antihistamine.*
>
> ANNE, MUM OF HANNAH AND EDWARD

During an allergic reaction, the skin is the most common part of the body affected. Hives – a red, lumpy itchy rash – is the most common skin symptom. The skin may also become swollen. The lips and eyelids may swell and the skin can become itchy and red and eczema may develop or become worse.

> *During weaning Hunter turned a bright red colour around his mouth when eating fish for the first time (cod mixed with a cheese sauce). The second time he had fish the red colour lasted much longer (I remember my dad saying that Hunter was 'not right'). On the third occasion Hunter turned red, and strange red welts appeared all over his face and upper body. He also vomited.*
>
> EMMA, MUM OF HUNTER

In an allergic reaction, the stomach and bowel may also be affected. An itchy mouth, stomach ache, nausea, vomiting and diarrhoea can all occur. These symptoms so far are not in themselves dangerous. They should be treated promptly with an antihistamine, which will stop the reaction progressing. Antihistamines can be prescribed or bought over the counter. There are specific antihistamine liquids that are suitable for children over one year. The dose is specified on the pack according to your child's age. There are ones that have longer-lasting effects such as Zirtek (active ingredient cetirizine) and ones that act for a shorter time such as Piriton (active ingredient chlorphenamine maleate). They should be given if your child has been exposed to an allergen. If your child is sick within 20 minutes of taking the antihistamine, a second dose should be given. Keep a close eye on your child for further symptoms.

Caution: Always read the labels and check with your doctor prior to using antihistamines for your child, especially if she is under one year old.

Non-life-threatening symptoms of an allergic reaction

The symptoms listed below are not life-threatening if experienced in isolation:

- Runny nose
- Diarrhoea
- Stomach pain
- Blocked nose
- Itching
- Red or itchy eyes
- Nausea or sickness
- Itchy mouth
- Lip swelling
- Odd taste in the mouth
- Flushed, red or swollen skin
- Hives
- Eczema flare

If your child has eaten or drunk a food that they are allergic to, then the symptoms in the list above should tell you that an allergic reaction is occurring. During the reaction, stay with your child and keep a close eye on her. Watch her breathing, and look for signs of tiredness and skin colour changes. If there is a worsening in any of these, the symptoms listed above or if any symptoms from the list opposite occur, then treatment with adrenaline is needed (see page 118), as discussed below. If you have an autoinjector, use it immediately. If this occurs then you must call '999' and state that your child is having an anaphylactic reaction.

Symptoms of an allergic reaction that are or may soon become life-threatening

Each symptom listed below on its own may indicate a more life-threatening reaction.

- Throat tightness
- Wheezing
- Shortness of breath
- Repetitive coughing
- Difficulty breathing
- High-pitched noises when breathing
- Changes in voice or cry – hoarseness
- Turning pale or bluish
- Tongue swelling
- Difficulty swallowing
- Low blood pressure
- Fainting
- Chest pain
- Dizziness
- Feeling of impending doom (older children)

At Easter 2010 (the boys were around 16 months old), Cameron had anaphylaxis... I went to work and had a call from the boys' nanny... to say Cameron had been sick as she was walking them back from dropping her children at school and she thought he might be choking. By the time I got home Cameron was having real difficulty breathing. I dialled 999 and an ambulance arrived within minutes. Still working on the choking assumption, they decided to take us in as he was clearly struggling. In the ambulance he became very red. When we got to A&E we were taken straight through. As we were walking down the corridors to the children's hospital Cameron suddenly went pale and limp in my arms – we ran the rest of the way. Cameron was injected with drugs – I don't know what, antihistamines I guess – and made a huge recovery quite quickly... After that we were given EpiPens and had the allergy testing with blood tests a little later as outpatients.

EMMA, MUM OF CAMERON AND DILLON

During a food-allergic reaction, symptoms differ and their order of appearance may vary. The reaction can be frightening enough but the appearance of symptoms is variable, which can make it difficult to recognise a potentially dangerous reaction. In people who have had a previous anaphylactic episode, there is a significant risk of recurrence. Avoidance of the allergen is the best way to prevent subsequent anaphylaxis but despite your best efforts to avoid the allergen, there is always a risk of accidental exposure.

Mild symptoms that do not progress to other areas of the body are usually not considered life-threatening anaphylaxis (for example, only a skin rash or only an itchy mouth). When breathing or blood circulation is affected, however, the allergic reaction is life-threatening anaphylaxis.

Anaphylaxis and What to Do

When your child is diagnosed with a food allergy, one of the most important things to discuss with your doctor is recognising and treating future reactions. However careful you are, these will happen from time to time and you need to be prepared. Although the majority of reactions are mild, a severe reaction is always possible. In a large study of children with milk allergy, every year 40 per cent of the children had an accidental reaction although only 10 per cent of these were severe (with no deaths). In nut allergy, around 20 per cent of children will have an accidental reaction each year.

Your doctor should discuss with you whether you should just be carrying antihistamines with you or whether there is an increased risk of severe reactions and therefore advise carrying adrenaline injectors. It is essential that you are given a written emergency treatment plan (nursery or school will need this) and that you are trained to know when as well as how to use the adrenaline injector (see page 118). The sooner adrenaline is administered during an anaphylactic reaction, the more rapid the recovery and better the outcome for your child – this is why children are given these to carry with them rather than waiting to get to hospital. As a parent you will be encouraged to use the autoinjector as soon as there is any sign of anaphylaxis, such as difficulty breathing, wheezing, stridor (see page 5), persistent cough or a hoarse voice, or if your child becomes pale, floppy or unresponsive.

As the parent of an allergic child, you will also be told by the healthcare professionals that if you are wondering whether your child's reaction is severe enough to warrant the use of their autoinjector, then this is probably the right time to administer it. That is good advice to pass on to any of your child's carers. If you aren't sure, use it.

In a severe allergic reaction, the priority is to give intramuscular adrenaline via an autoinjector (EpiPen or Jext). If you are alone with your child, give the adrenaline before you call 999. If there is somebody with you, they can call 999 while you give the adrenaline. State that you have given an AAI to your child to treat anaphylaxis for known food allergy. The paramedics will assess your child and take her to hospital, with you, to either continue treatment or monitor her for a while.

After this, asthma inhalers can be given via a spacer device, if your child is asthmatic as can antihistamine if your child is able to swallow.

Your child may need a second injection of adrenaline after 10–15 minutes if she has not made a clear improvement and the ambulance has not yet arrived.

During an allergic reaction, your child should be placed in the lying position and the adrenaline autoinjector (AAI) administered. Do not try to sit or stand her up or get her to move around as this will cause a drop in blood pressure.

EpiPen and Jext Autoinjectors

EpiPen, Jext and Emerade are all adrenaline autoinjectors (AAIs) that are used for the injection of the drug adrenaline or epinephrine, the first-line treatment for life-threatening allergic reactions. They have different names and there are adult and child versions of these autoinjectors. They provide different drug doses, but they essentially all look similar and do the same job. AAIs are rarely needed in a child who is under one year of age. However, if your child is felt to be at high risk of a severe reaction, they must be referred to a paediatric allergy specialist who can then prescribe an AAI at eight months old, at the doctor's discretion, if the risk of anaphylaxis is high.

How to use an adrenaline auto injector (AAI)

It is very important that you are taught in person how to use the AAI by the healthcare professional who prescribes it for your child. In addition to this teaching, your child's AAI will come with instructions, so please read these carefully and have a look at the AAI websites (see page 260) for a recap on its use.

To give the AAI:

- Remove the AAI from its outer packaging.
- Remove the safety cap at the flat end.
- There is no need to remove your child's clothing.
- Hold your child securely and tightly, as close to a lying position as possible, if she is not unconscious. A child who is not unconscious may well struggle and fight, especially when the AAI is administered. It is important that you hold her and particularly her leg still while the AAI is given.
- If she has lost consciousness or is drowsy, place her on the floor on her side and kneel beside her.
- Follow the method that the healthcare professionals have taught you to inject the AAI.
- A click should be heard, indicating that the adrenaline is being administered.
- Hold the pen in place for a slow count of 10.
- Holding your child, remove the AAI carefully and place it somewhere out of the way.
- Massage your child's leg for 10 seconds.

It is so important to recognise that you cannot delay giving your child the AAI. It does take courage and many parents are fearful of hurting their child but it is no worse than any other injection. In the situation of an anaphylactic reaction, there should be no delay in giving the AAI. It is a matter of life and death and needs to be given immediately. Any delay could affect the outcome for your child.

The decision to prescribe an AAI

The AAI will be prescribed by a doctor, usually your child's allergy specialist. While adrenaline is the most effective treatment for severe allergic reactions, its prompt administration requires patients to be carrying their own adrenaline injectors. Prescriptions of these have risen dramatically over the past two decades and most classrooms in the country will now have had a child who carries one. However, it remains extremely difficult to decide which child should carry these. On the one hand, IgE mediated allergic reactions are inherently unpredictable and many cases of severe reactions happen in people who had previously only had mild reactions. Prescribing everyone at risk of anaphylaxis an AAI therefore seems an attractive idea. On the other hand, this approach is enormously draining on healthcare resources – severe reactions are rare and the overwhelming majority of AAIs are never used, simply going out of date. More concerning, however, is that over-prescription of AAIs leads to a failure to focus adequately on children who have the highest risk of severe reactions. Most people prescribed AAIs do not carry them and of those that do, many are unable to use them. It would therefore make more sense to select children with the highest risk for anaphylaxis and ensure that they and their families are properly trained to use their AAIs and that they ensure they always carry them. This is the preferred approach of most doctors but selecting high-risk children is also challenging. In truth, the decision as to whether to prescribe AAIs is very much an individual one requiring discussion between the doctor and family. Being prescribed an AAI can significantly alter quality of life – in some families they act as a 'safety blanket'; in others they create heightened anxiety. Every family has its own approach to risk and hence there will never be precise protocol on which child should carry an AAI.

There are some international guidelines for doctors to use to help decision-making. These are widely in agreement that any child with

IgE mediated food allergy who has had a previous anaphylaxis or has concurrent asthma, should have an AAI. Of course, this means proper training in when and how to use it, and a written emergency plan. You must take the AAI everywhere that your child goes and eventually when they are old enough, your child will have to take on some of the responsibility for carrying their own AAI. Other risk factors that should influence the decision are the presence of allergies most likely to cause severe reactions, such as nut allergy, being distant from medical care or having had reactions to tiny quantities of allergen (although it remains debatable as to whether this increases the risk of severe reactions).

Another debate centres on how many AAIs need to be carried – some say two, others one and there are sound arguments on both sides, again in the context that few AAIs are ever used. While some children do need a second dose of adrenaline, as the first has not been effective (or the device is not correctly administered), in a UK setting there is almost always emergency medical care on hand by the time this is necessary. Most children will have two sets of AAIs – one to be left at school and the other to take around with them everywhere else. Some schools (mirroring what is happening in the US) are starting to have a set of AAIs that can be used on any child, rather than having multiple sets from different children.

In summary, whether to have AAIs and how many to carry is a very individual decision that needs to be made with your doctor. What is clear, however, is that simply being prescribed an AAI is never enough. You need proper training, with the right supporting emergency plan and must carry the injector everywhere.

AAIs do expire, so it's a good idea to register your AAI with a website that will email or text you a reminder. There are a few different websites that offer this service for free (see the Resources section on page 260). Repeat prescriptions are available from your GP.

Possible side-effects

There are some side-effects to giving an adrenaline into the muscle, the most common being an increased heart rate, sweating, nausea and vomiting, shakiness, headache, apprehension, nervousness or anxiety. However, these side-effects will usually go away quickly, especially if your child is able to rest. Adrenaline is safe when injected via an AAI and there is no risk of being sorry you gave it – only that it may not have been necessary.

Looking after and using an AAI

The AAI should be kept at room temperature (25°C/77°F), which is worth bearing in mind on a hot day or when travelling to a hot country abroad. There are bags available specifically for carrying AAIs, which are also designed to keep them at the right temperature.

The Resources section at the back of this book (see page 258) provides details of where these can be purchased. Once you have given the AAI, it is not reusable.

Unfortunately, a large proportion of children who are prescribed AAIs do not carry them with them and even when they do, their carers are not able to use them properly. It is important to remember that reactions will happen when you least expect and you need to be prepared in advance for what you will do. Don't wait until your child is struggling to breathe to start reading the instructions on the AAI.

My son was diagnosed at the age of one, after having a bite of a peanut butter sandwich. He ended up in Accident and Emergency and Intensive Therapy Unit overnight.

ERICA, MUM OF EVAN

The three times we used the EpiPen... Kobe [had] started to have asthma issues – he couldn't breathe and was coughing and sneezing. The first time this happened I waited too long, we were so new at this and didn't really know what to do. He turned white, unresponsive and was panting slowly. We used the EpiPen and he instantly was fine. It was almost like whatever it was jumped out of him (crazy sounding, I know). We called 999 each time and the ambulance was very helpful.

BRANDY, MUM OF KOBE

Anaphylaxis typically appears as described above by Brandy, Kobe's mum. It is a rapid appearance of the symptoms above. Your child will eat the food, get hives and swelling around the mouth which spread and then the difficulty breathing starts. In this situation, the AAI must always be given and an ambulance called. However, severe reactions are not always typical and in these cases, when in doubt, the AAI should always be given.

I didn't hear the word 'anaphylaxis' until one of the specialist nurses came to see me much later on as we were in the waiting room to go home. It still hadn't occurred to me that was what had happened. I remember being shocked – I knew the boys had an allergy but it had never occurred to me that anaphylaxis was a possibility. At that point the seriousness of what had happened to my baby boy hit me and I was terrified. I was sent home with one or two EpiPens. It was weeks later that I remembered that a friend had been round making Easter eggs for her cousins with chocolate buttons. I think one must have fallen under the washing machine and Cameron found it and ate it.

I have now researched as much as I possibly can about anaphylaxis. Cameron didn't have really obvious signs save for the difficulty breathing and flushed skin. He didn't swell up and didn't have hives around his mouth. His reaction was delayed by at least an hour, possibly more. I think we were so lucky – that I got home from work quickly, that the ambulance came quickly and that the lovely registrar noticed the hives. I dread to think what would have happened if we hadn't got medical attention so quickly. I hadn't had any training or advice on signs of anaphylaxis, we hadn't had any testing for allergies and I had no idea how serious it could be.

EMMA, MUM OF CAMERON AND DILLON

My first experience of Zach having a severe reaction was when he was 19 months old. At a friend's house he ate a small bit of a 'free from' crumpet. I didn't think to check the packet until the last minute and it contained egg white. It was a strange experience. He didn't react straight away, in fact nothing happened for about 30 minutes. In that time, I started to think that maybe he was no longer allergic. Then he very rapidly deteriorated. He began to sneeze repeatedly and scratch his nose. His nose and eyes became swollen and patches became raised and red on his arms and legs. He was crying, hot and red, so I took him outside. At that point he stopped crying and became drowsy. His eyes were rolling backwards and he felt a bit limp. I put him in his pushchair because I thought he might be tired. I quickly realised what a bad decision that was so picked him up again, and jiggled him around and shouted at him to stay awake while I ran back to my friend's house. I didn't know what to do so I called my medic husband and he told me to give him a large dose of Piriton. My friend ran to a pharmacy and that's what we did. Zach then fell asleep on me for an hour. When he woke up, his skin had gone down, but he stood up and turned deep blue around his mouth and nose. His whole body began to shake and he was very cold. We wrapped him up, but he was okay and was smiling and wanted to play. We gave him more Piriton and the worst of the reaction was over. Before that happened, I thought I was quite calm in a crisis. I am used to emergency situations from working in the NHS. However, when it happened to Zach, I didn't know what to do and it took me ages to realise what was happening. I should have given him the EpiPen and I should have been carrying an antihistamine with me, as he was clearly having an anaphylactic reaction. No matter how prepared I thought that I was, when it happened to my son, I was frightened and not prepared at all.

This experience taught me that it can be difficult for parents to know when a reaction is severe and what to do about it. However, it is important for you, your child and childcare providers to be clear about what symptoms can occur during an allergic reaction and which ones are dangerous and require emergency treatment with an adrenaline autoinjector. If you are unsure whether your child is having an anaphylactic reaction, but she has the symptoms, always give the AAI and call an ambulance.

After my first experience of Zach's anaphylaxis, the paediatrician asked me if I had been scared. When I replied that I had, he said 'Good, you should be. It's meant to be scary'.

The next few chapters will discuss aspects of the allergic march, the progression through the different atopic illnesses that will commonly affect children with food allergies. As we know, allergies have increased dramatically in the Western world over the past few decades. Recent research has shown that an incredible 40 per cent of UK children have at least one allergic problem. This includes conditions such as eczema, asthma and food allergy, although the most common allergic problem is allergic rhinitis or hay fever.

CHAPTER 9
Eczema

Eczema, particularly in babies, is linked with a risk of developing food allergies. The more severe your baby's eczema is and the earlier in life that they develop eczema, the more likely they are to develop food allergies. A baby with severe eczema before three months of age is very likely to suffer from IgE mediated food allergies. Children with eczema and food allergy are very likely to get later respiratory problems.

Until Zach was referred to a dermatologist at eight months old, he had suffered itchy, dry skin with red raw patches that looked like burn marks. He had also had blistering skin infections that looked dreadful. He had been extremely uncomfortable and unsettled. Once referred to the dermatologist, he was diagnosed with severe eczema and the link was made with possible food allergies. Allergy blood tests were carried out, which came back as positive for food allergies. The dermatology team gave us a skincare regime, which started us on the road to recovery for his skin.

It is now estimated that 'atopic' or 'allergic' eczema affects almost 20 per cent of children. Atopic eczema (also known as atopic dermatitis) is a chronic itchy skin condition that most commonly develops in early childhood. Eczema tends to be variable, with children suffering from dry skin, which flares up with sore patches from time to time, often for no apparent reason. Fortunately, for most children eczema is relatively mild, although still irritating. However, for a smaller proportion of children, eczema can be more severe and continuous, having a significant impact on a child's quality of life as well as that of their parents. In a recent survey of parents of children with eczema by the National Eczema Society, one in six mums said they would consider having no more children if they too would suffer from eczema. The GP may manage your child's eczema but sometimes a referral to a dermatologist is required.

Symptoms of Eczema

The most common symptoms of eczema are dry, itchy skin and rashes on the face, inside the elbows and behind the knees, and on the hands and feet. Itching is the most significant symptom of eczema. Scratching and rubbing in response to itching irritates the skin, increases inflammation and actually increases the itchiness, leading to a vicious 'itch-scratch' cycle. As well as the most common symptoms, it is also important to know the exacerbating factors of eczema. Medical treatments are mainly symptomatic relief with the aim of reversing and preventing the problems, such as skin infections that can result from eczema. These treatments include moisture replacement, treatment of infection and lessening the immune response. In other words, the doctor is trying to heal the skin and prevent exacerbations. To meet these aims, a solid skincare regime needs to be established, in conjunction with you the parent, and it needs to be rigidly adhered to.

Skincare regimes are written by the dermatology team, which includes the dermatologist and the nurse specialists. The regimes are personalised to your child and should include a contact name and number for further support. The skincare regime will help, along with the avoidance of substances that lead to skin irritation and trigger the immune system and the itch-scratch cycle. It is therefore vital to know what these triggers are and it is important for you to note any changes in your child's skin condition in response to treatment, and to be persistent in identifying the treatment that seems to work best, as well as in identifying the triggers that make it worse. Take extra care or avoid using any products on the skin that are perfumed or not prescribed and be careful with detergents and fabric conditioners, as products can often contain an allergen and go unidentified. In essence, think through anything that will come into contact with your child's skin and make it as skin-friendly and non-irritant as possible.

Common Skin Irritants

- Wool or synthetic fibres
- Soaps and detergents
- Some perfumes and cosmetics
- Substances such as chlorine, mineral oil or solvents
- Dust or sand
- Cigarette smoke

As well as the irritants listed above, the following factors may worsen the symptoms of eczema.

- Allergies to food, pollen, mould, dust mites or animals
- Cold and dry air in the winter
- Being run down with a cold or flu
- Dry skin
- Emotional stress
- You may find that when your child has a cold, a poor night's sleep, is teething and so on his skin also flares up as his body responds to the additional stress. Chicken pox in particular can cause nasty eczema flares

When eczema occurs during infancy and childhood, it affects each child differently in terms of both onset and severity of symptoms. In babies, eczema typically begins around 6–12 weeks of age. It may first appear around the cheeks and chin as a patchy facial rash, which can progress to red, scaling, oozing skin. Once your child becomes more mobile and begins crawling, exposed areas, such as the inner and outer parts of the arms and legs, may also be affected. Your child may be restless and irritable because of the itching and discomfort.

> *The first symptom on both boys was eczema. First of all patches on the arms, then on the cheeks (developed in the same place on the same day in both boys... freaky twin stuff!). By the time the GP got on to it and we had a referral to the dermatologist (lots of visits later with me feeling more and more like a neurotic mother) both boys were raw and weeping over at least 50 per cent of their bodies and faces.*
>
> EMMA, MUM OF CAMERON AND DILLON

In childhood, the rash tends to occur behind the knees and inside the elbows; on the sides of the neck; around the mouth; and on the wrists, ankles and hands. Often, the rash begins with tiny spots that become hard and scaly when scratched. The skin around the lips may be inflamed, and constant licking of the area may lead to small, painful cracks in the skin around the mouth.

Skincare Regime
● ●

Your child's skincare regime is vital to heal the skin, keep it healthy, stop infections and further damage and, most importantly, to enhance your child's quality of life. Developing and sticking with a daily skincare routine is critical to preventing flares. This can be time consuming and difficult with a young child but it is essential. I incorporated massage into the routine, along with play and my own skincare regime so that Zach could copy and make it a normal part of his life. With perseverance and patience the daily routines did become easier.

Moisturising

It is important to keep your child's skin well moisturised in order to keep it healthy. Your child's skin can become dried out as a result of regular and frequent baths or showers or from swimming very often. While bathing is vital, especially when your child has eczema, and swimming is part and parcel of life, a few changes to your routine can help to preserve or replace the moisture within your child's skin. For example, it may be worth adding a bath additive such as an oil to help counteract the drying effects of bathing. Change the products that you use in the bath as well as the cleaning agents so that they are non-abrasive and gentle on your baby's skin (see page 132). Do not use soap or other detergents.

It became clear why Levi's skin had become so bad and why he had been wheezy after baths. The dermatologist realised that the bath oil he had been prescribed for his skin actually contained nut oil... it was why his skin was becoming worse not better. The amazing thing was that as soon as we ceased using the oil and changed his milk his skin recovered to almost perfect in a matter of about a week or two.

BEV, MUM OF LEVI

Bathing

To add moisture to your child's skin, use an emollient wash in the bath, rather than soap, as soap is drying to the skin. The most effective, such as Hydromol and Epaderm, which are paraffin-based, can be bought or prescribed. A lukewarm bath helps to cleanse and moisturise the skin without drying it excessively. After bathing, allow your child to air-dry the skin, or pat their skin dry gently (avoiding rubbing or brisk drying), and then apply an emollient to seal in the water that has been absorbed into the skin during bathing. A lubricant increases the rate of healing and establishes a barrier against further drying and irritation. Lotions that have a high water or alcohol content evaporate more quickly, and alcohol may cause stinging. Therefore, they generally are not the best choice. Ointments work better at healing the skin and keeping moisture in but feel greasier. Any products used on your child's skin should be unperfumed so as not to irritate the skin further.

Swimming

When going swimming, it is a good idea to dress your child in a full-body swimsuit, having covered their skin in the prescription emollient such as Hydromol first. This will act as a barrier between their skin and the water to minimise any drying effects. After swimming, try to ensure that your child always showers well to remove chlorine and then moisturise as soon as possible before dressing. If your child has particularly poor skin at any time, then it may be worth missing a week or two of swimming to allow time for the skin to heal.

Avoiding infection

Another key to protecting and restoring the skin is taking steps to avoid skin infections. Skin infections occur where skin has broken down, allowing bacteria in. Signs of skin infection include discoloration, tiny pus-filled bumps, oozing cracks, sores on the skin or crusty yellow blisters. If symptoms of a skin infection develop, visit your GP as soon as possible to get the right treatment quickly. At home, to tackle infections, first bath your child in warm water to remove crusts and pat the skin dry. Stick to your child's skincare regime and follow the instructions on the antibiotic ointment or oral antibiotic medicine that will have been provided for your child's specific skin infection.

Reducing irritation

Irritated skin leads to itching and then scratching which, as we have already mentioned, leads to more irritation. Bear in mind that itching is a particular problem when your child is asleep because conscious control of scratching is lost and you are not there to stop them. To reduce skin irritation, use cotton clothing and bedding, mild detergents and mild or prescription soaps and shampoos. Keep your child's fingernails short, the bedroom cool and try putting mitts on his hands at night-time to prevent excessive scratching and rubbing. We used to swaddle Zach at night-time and put him in mitts to prevent the scratching. I didn't know if I was being helpful or making his skin more irritated. Either way, by the morning he had always wriggled free and caused a new scratch on his face.

Caution: If you suspect food allergy, check ingredients of detergents as well as soaps, and washing-up liquids, as some contain milk products. Only use non-biological detergents.

Immune Response

To reduce the immune response, in other words, to reduce the sore, inflamed areas of skin, steroid creams and other non-steroidal medications may be prescribed. These help to settle the immune response and reduce inflammation. Long-term steroid use can cause skin thinning. However, when used carefully, under the direction of a specialised doctor, steroid creams are both effective and safe. Under-treated eczema can lead to skin damage. Antihistamines can also be used to reduce itchiness and sedating versions can be helpful at night. If your child is under one, antihistamines can only be used on prescription. Piriton is fine at a dose of 1mg but only on prescription from your doctor.

Zach was prescribed a strong steroid by the dermatologist. However, every time I ordered a repeat prescription from the GP or went to collect it from the chemist, I was given a lecture about the extreme seriousness of giving steroids to a small baby and was asked if I was sure I knew what I was doing. The quick answer to that question, quite clearly, was no I didn't, but I followed what the dermatologist told me and learnt to ignore and smile at the other comments. When Zach was older and we had an appointment with an allergy specialist, he told me the importance of the use of strong steroids and that, while they do have their risks if used inappropriately for long periods, if severe eczema is left under-treated, the risk of damage to the skin can be far greater.

Do not confuse the many side-effects of taking high-dose steroids by mouth, with those of using steroid creams on the skin – they are very different. For those where steroids are needed on an extended basis, you may be offered a calcineurin inhibitor cream – these are newer and act in a similar way to steroids but without the skin-thinning side-effect.

Before trying any treatment, always seek medical advice first. As previously discussed, the dermatologist will have a team of professionals working together. A personal skincare plan, skin evaluation sheets and nurse specialists are extremely valuable especially in the early days of managing skin conditions. That support and management is vital.

Essentials

- Give lukewarm baths.
- Bath in non-soap replacer. Visit your GP to get this on prescription.
- After patting dry, apply steroid to the sore bits. Then wait 30 minutes before using moisturiser.
- Follow a skincare regime for your child.
- Use steroids if and when prescribed and follow directions for timing and duration of use.
- Do not apply steroids just after moisturisers as steroids create a barrier over the skin and stop the moisturisers from working.
- Keep your child's fingernails short.
- Select soft cotton fabrics when choosing clothing and bedding.
- Use washing powder, washing liquids and fabric conditioners intended for sensitive skin.
- Consider using antihistamines to promote sleep and reduce scratching at night. Always seek medical advice first.
- Keep your child cool, especially at night.
- Avoid situations where overheating occurs.
- Learn to recognise skin infections and seek treatment promptly.
- Attempt to distract your child with activities to keep her from scratching.
- Identify and remove irritants and allergens.
- Ask for a referral to a dermatologist if you are in any doubt or feel that your child's skin is being poorly managed.

Eczema and Food Allergy

Eczema may flare up for a variety of reasons such as skin infections, irritants (such as abrasive clothing or sweating), viral infections as well as numerous other factors. Many parents also worry that their child's diet may be one of the causes of their child's eczema. In fact, studies have shown that 75 per cent of mothers have made changes to their child's diet in order to try to improve their eczema. Many doctors are sceptical that there is any value in such dietary manipulation, which may place the child at risk of missing out on essential nutrients, as well as resulting in the considerable hardship that careful avoidance of any specific food will lead to. However, the understanding of the possible role of food allergy in eczema has improved considerably and it is becoming increasingly clear that in some children, identifying and excluding problem foods can have a significant impact on eczema. Identifying the correct foods in the correct children still requires considerable expertise. If you are concerned about your child's eczema and suspect a link with food, it is important to raise your concerns with your family doctor or paediatrician rather than experimenting yourself.

Where there is eczema, there is often food allergy

There appears to have been a large increase in food allergy over recent decades, although this has been less well documented than the increase in other allergic disease. Peanut allergy, for example, has tripled in just over a decade and now affects almost 1 in 50 children in the English-speaking world. As we have discussed, food allergies can be very broadly divided into immediate allergies (see page 4), which lead to immediate symptoms such as hives, wheeziness and, in severe cases, anaphylaxis (a life-threatening allergic reaction) and those which cause more delayed symptoms (see page 5). Immediate reactions are usually quite obvious when they occur as they produce obvious symptoms very soon after the food is eaten and can also be confirmed with special allergy tests. Delayed reactions involve a different part of the immune system and may be very tricky to diagnose, as symptoms may occur many hours after the food is eaten, and as yet there are no reliable tests to confirm which food is the problem. Continuing to eat a food where there is a delayed allergy can lead to persistence and worsening of the eczema while removing it can improve the eczema. Eczema is thus associated with immediate food allergies, delayed food allergies or both, which is why the relationship often seems so complex.

Eczema and immediate food allergies

There is a very close relationship between eczema and immediate food allergies. Almost all of the children in an allergy clinic who have immediate food allergies will either have eczema or will have had it during the first year of life. This strongly suggests that eczema may have a causative role in food allergies and this is currently the subject of a lot of interest in the scientific world. There is also a clear relationship between the age that the eczema first appeared, how severe it is and the likelihood of having one of these types of food allergy. The earlier that eczema starts and the more severe that it is, the greater the chance of having immediate food allergies. Studies have shown that children with severe eczema that started before three months of age are at particular risk (and most will have a food allergy), while those who did not develop eczema until they were over one year old were much less likely to have a food allergy.

Most immediate food allergy is caused by a relatively small number of different foods (see Chapters 2 and 3).

Eczema and delayed food allergies

The link between delayed food allergies and eczema has only become apparent more recently. The suggestion that a child could be eating something regularly in their diet, which is worsening their eczema, is still not taken seriously by some doctors. While most children with eczema will not be suffering from delayed food allergies, correctly identifying problem foods in the right children can lead to significant improvements in eczema and thus reduce the reliance on steroid creams to keep the skin under control. Research in this area has suggested that it is milk, egg, soya and wheat that are the most likely culprits and again it is those children whose eczema starts early in infancy and is severe that are most likely to respond to dietary changes. However, the allergy tests used to diagnose immediate allergies (such as skin prick tests or a blood test known as specific IgE) are of much less value in delayed allergies.

Many companies offer food testing over the internet to identify foods that may worsen eczema. These tests offer at-home finger prick blood tests or hair samples, which are then sent off in the post. However, there is no evidence to support these and they can often lead to completely pointless food exclusions. These tests are not used by allergists or dermatologists. While these tests appear to offer a quick and easy solution, there is currently no substitute for evaluation by an experienced doctor or dietician. After taking a detailed history, they may advise the complete elimination of specific foods and carefully evaluate the results. Even if excluding a particular food does appear to help, it is essential that an attempt to reintroduce the food is made (which would be expected to lead to a worsening of the eczema) in order to confirm that the food is a problem.

Clues that your child's eczema may be related to food

When evaluating a child with eczema, your doctor will pick up on certain clues that raise the possibility of food being a problem. As mentioned earlier, it is children with moderate to severe eczema that starts before six months of age that are most likely to have a food allergy. Milk is the most common allergen.

- Moderate to severe eczema.
- Eczema that first appeared at less than six months of age.
- Family history of allergies, such as asthma, eczema and hay fever.
- Eczema does not respond as well as expected to treatment, such as with steroid creams.
- Gastrointestinal symptoms such as colic, reflux, diarrhoea or poor weight gain.
- Worsening of eczema after meals including breast milk (think about what you had eaten earlier and consider keeping a food diary to pick up any consistent patterns).
- Presence of one food allergy – if your child has an obvious allergy to one food, consider if another is also causing problems

Caution: It is important to remember that food allergy and diet often plays no role in eczema and while it is necessary for you to keep an open mind, it is never a good idea to restrict your child's diet without good reason. Any restriction must be under the supervision of a doctor or dietician. If removing a food from your child's diet does not seem to help and reintroducing it does not make things worse, then it is very unlikely to be a problem and should not be further restricted.

What to Do if You Suspect that Food is a Problem

If you suspect that your child has an immediate food allergy or that something she is eating is making her eczema worse, then you should discuss this with your doctor. A food exclusion or trial or allergy tests may be recommended. Most large hospitals have a paediatric or dermatology department where one of the doctors has an interest in allergy and a few large teaching hospitals have specialist paediatric allergists.

Fortunately, most children grow out of their eczema by later childhood and many common food allergies, such as milk and egg, are also often outgrown. It is therefore important that, if a diagnosis of food allergy is made, your child should still receive ongoing follow-up care to check for the possibility that the food could be safely introduced.

CHAPTER 10

Allergic Rhinitis

Allergic rhinitis is a swelling of the inside lining of the nose as a result of an allergy to something in the air. The most common type is seasonal allergic rhinitis (better known as hay fever), which is the result of an allergy to grass or tree pollen. Symptoms may last all year round if they are caused by a 'perennial' allergen such as dust mites, or cat or dog fur.

Signs and Symptoms of Allergic Rhinitis

- Itching of the nose, ears, mouth or throat
- Sneezing episodes
- Thin, clear runny mucus discharge from the nose
- Blocked nose
- Sinus headache
- Feeling of blocked ears
- Mouth breathing or snoring
- Dry cough
- Frequent throat clearing
- Sleep disturbance
- Daytime tiredness

Typical features of allergic rhinitis, as shown above, are sneezing, a blocked, itchy and runny nose, together with itchy eyes (allergic conjunctivitis). However, in more severe cases it may cause disturbed sleep, lethargy, sinusitis and glue ear. While often being thought of as a problem of adulthood, allergic rhinitis is becoming increasingly common in children, affecting around 10 per cent of 6 to 7-year-olds. As allergic rhinitis has become more common over time, it is also affecting increasingly younger children. It is particularly common in children with asthma. Around 50–80 per cent of asthmatics also suffer from allergic rhinitis.

In allergic rhinitis, as with food allergy, the swelling and symptoms are caused by an immunoglobulin E (IgE) mediated immune response to specific allergens such as pollen, mould, animal dander and dust mites. It is again important that you are able to give a clear account to your doctor of what your child's symptoms are and most importantly what seems to cause them and when they are triggered.

Although symptoms of allergic rhinitis are not life-threatening, they can have detrimental effects on the physical, psychological and social aspects of your child's life. Allergic rhinitis can significantly decrease quality of life and this is often under-recognised by healthcare professionals and non-sufferers alike.

Symptoms of allergic rhinitis and the associated effect on quality of sleep have significant effects on a child's ability to perform well at school. Even uncomplicated allergic rhinitis may be associated with reduced ability to learn. This is a particular concern for older children because the timing of public examinations coincides with the grass pollen season. A study comparing adolescents' examination performance during 'mock' examinations (conducted in winter) with formal examinations in spring/ summer, revealed that having current symptomatic allergic rhinitis was associated with a remarkable 50 per cent increase in the risk of dropping an exam grade between winter and summer. Frustratingly, while even severe allergic rhinitis can be effectively treated, many patients often receive bad advice, resulting in unnecessary suffering.

Effective Management of Allergic Rhinitis

The most effective way to reduce symptoms of allergic rhinitis is by avoiding the problem allergen. When it is unclear what the problem allergen is, allergy testing can be very helpful. The most common cause of year-round symptoms (or those that are worse in the winter) is dust mite faeces. Dust mites are tiny, spider-like creatures, invisible to the naked eye. They like warm, moist environments such as bedding and soft furnishing. They eat human skin particles and it is their droppings that cause allergic problems. If allergy to dust mites is causing allergic rhinitis (or asthma or eczema), then reducing exposure to them should help. The most useful measure is getting special covers for the mattress and bedding. These prevent the faecal particles getting up the nose while sleeping. It is essential to get the right covers, which are properly tested as being effective. A good example would be AllerGuard (www.allerguard.co.uk) or those approved by the Allergy UK 'Seal of Approval' as this means they have been rigorously tested. Other measures include reducing the amount of soft toys and furnishings, and regular damp dusting. Replacing carpet with hard floors is sometimes helpful but the effect is quite limited.

Last summer, when he was aged seven, Felix started getting really itchy eyes in spring and summer. The GP said it was hay fever and prescribed loratadine, which worked. We went to the GP last week for a new prescription, and I asked if we should allergy test but he said, if the antihistamine works then there is your answer! So his symptoms are mainly itchy eyes, sometimes a bit snuffly. It is definitely worse on sunny days and when he is outside, in the garden, on the school play field. etc. If I don't give him the medicine (on a sunny day), I generally get called into school to give it so I am much better at remembering!

EMILY, MUM OF FELIX, FINN AND LEO

Unfortunately, with hay fever there is much less that can be done to avoid pollen. Pollen filters in cars, wrap-around sunglasses and nightly hair washes, to prevent transfer of pollen from the hair to the pillow, all may help.

Medication

In most cases, allergen avoidance measures are not enough and medication may be required. Over-the-counter antihistamines are useful but it is essential to ensure that a long-acting, non-sedating one is used otherwise the drowsy side-effects can make your child feel even worse. Cetirizine (Zirtek) or loratidine (Clarityn) are good choices. Beyond this, nasal sprays with tiny doses of steroids can be extremely effective. These need to be prescribed by your doctor.

For those with more severe allergic rhinitis, the combination of antihistamine and nasal spray may still not be enough and a referral to an allergy specialist is worth considering. Newer nasal sprays, containing both steroid and antihistamine (such as Dymista) are also effective and may be worth trying.

Desensitisation

An allergist can use allergy tests to confirm what the cause of the problem is and may also recommend desensitisation (also known as immunotherapy), as discussed in Chapter 12. This is a highly effective treatment that aims to reduce the allergic response, preventing the symptoms in the nose and eyes from happening in the first place (as opposed to trying to suppress symptoms with antihistamines and steroids). To achieve this, your child's immune system is gradually exposed to increasing amounts of the allergen, such as grass pollen. There are a number of very attractive benefits to this type of treatment. Firstly, it reduces symptoms and reliance on medication without using drugs. Furthermore, because immunotherapy treatment changes the underlying cause of the allergy, after three years, treatment can be stopped, but the effect continues for years afterwards. Children who have been desensitised have also been shown to be less likely to go on to develop asthma.

Desensitisation can be done by injection or using tablets or drops that are placed under the tongue. Both are safe, although there is a chance of having potential severe reactions to the injections and hence this needs to be done under very close supervision and is not really suited to those who already suffer from asthma. Both sorts of immunotherapy should be done under the supervision of an experienced doctor. Frustratingly, as there are so few trained allergists (particularly paediatric allergists) in the UK, while desensitisation treatments are used widely around the world, they have remained relatively inaccessible in the UK. There are UK centres that do carry it out, however, so if you are concerned about the severity of your child's allergic rhinitis, ask your GP to refer your child.

The summer before Zach turned four, he developed allergic rhinitis. It seemed to start overnight almost, with a constant sniff, running eyes, rubbing his nose and sneezing. He has been referred for desensitisation. He has been given an inhaler for coughing and signs of asthma and seems to be following the pattern of the allergic march. The desensitisation starts from around five years of age. It is hoped that desensitisation will prevent the worsening of asthma in Zach and therefore prevent worsening of his food allergic reactions.

The Link with Asthma

The link between allergic rhinitis and asthma is important. As mentioned there is a big overlap, with 50 per cent of children with allergic rhinitis developing asthma, while the majority of asthmatics have allergic rhinitis. The link becomes clearest in the summer when rising pollen counts lead to an increasing number of asthma attacks. The presence of allergic rhinitis symptoms has been clearly linked with loss of asthma control. Perhaps, most importantly, correctly recognising and treating rhinitis has been shown to reduce asthma attacks. In short, these conditions can't be considered in isolation. If your child has one of these, you need to be on the lookout for the other.

CHAPTER 11
Asthma

As part of the allergic march (see pages 11–12), children with food allergies are at a greater risk of developing asthma. Asthma is a condition that affects the airways, the tubes that carry air in and out of the lungs. When a person with asthma comes into contact with something that irritates their airways, this is called an asthma trigger.

When the airways become irritated, the muscles around the walls of the airways tighten so that the airways become narrower and the lining of the airways becomes swollen. Sometimes sticky mucus or phlegm builds up, which can further narrow the airways. The most common asthma trigger is an infection – simple coughs and colds – while others include cold air, exercise and tobacco smoke.

Symptoms of Asthma

- Coughing – particularly at night or with exercise
- Wheezing
- Shortness of breath
- Tightness in the chest

Asthma and Food Allergies

Asthma is a common problem for children with food allergy as they grow up, with 80 per cent of children with egg allergy going on to develop asthma and 70–75 per cent of those with nut allergy (see Allergy management in the Resources section page 253). It is extremely important that if your child develops asthma, the symptoms are spotted early and the management is optimal. This is because there is a link between asthma and the severity of food allergic reactions. If your child's asthma is poorly controlled, he has a greater risk of having a more severe, life-threatening reaction to his allergenic food. The link is also found the other way in that food allergies can trigger life-threatening asthma attacks. Either way, it is vitally important that both your child's food allergies and asthma are well controlled in order to minimise the severity of either.

Children with milk allergy are 10 times more likely to have a severe allergic reaction if they also have asthma, than those without asthma. Although death from food allergy is very rare, a high proportion of such fatal reactions occur in people with poorly controlled asthma because the breathing system is already suffering from the asthma and an anaphylactic reaction puts further strain on the breathing (see Resources section). Understanding why an allergic reaction may be mild on one occasion but devastating on another remains poor. However, there are certain risk factors for more severe reactions, the most important of which is the presence of asthma. Almost all fatal cases of anaphylaxis occur in asthmatics.

Management of Asthma
••

Early detection of the development of asthma is important. Therefore, your child needs to have regular reviews with his doctor who will be watching for the symptoms. If you suspect your child has any of the symptoms of asthma, always err on the side of caution. Discuss with your GP at the slightest concern about your child's breathing to get an early diagnosis and inhaler prescription to begin managing his symptoms.

Our GP was brilliant. Zach had a few nights of non-stop coughing and a bit of coughing in the day when he ran around. I took him to the GP who prescribed a salbutamol inhaler with spacer device to be used four times a day. We opted for the facemask rather than mouthpiece. Zach uses it well and his coughing is much better, allowing him to sleep.

If you have any concerns that your child's symptoms are not improving, revisit your GP until you feel that they are well controlled. Steroid inhalers, which prevent asthma attacks, can be prescribed as well as tablets for children with more severe asthma. It may be better to risk a degree of over-treating your child, than allow symptoms of poorly controlled asthma to go undetected or be poorly managed, as the risks to health are too great in the context of the food allergy.

With good asthma control your child will be free from symptoms. In a child too young to complain of symptoms, poor control can show itself by the presence of a night-time cough, wheezing or cough following known triggers (cold, exercise, allergens) and repeated hospital admissions. Peak flow monitoring where your child blows into a device that measures his breath, can be introduced at about five years old, depending on the child. Even if technique is initially poor, it may be beneficial to introduce the practice early on to encourage compliance later on.

If your child's asthma is not well controlled, and he needs to be given the reliever inhaler (usually blue) regularly (more than 3–4 times a week), then discuss this with your doctor. In the UK, there is a standard guideline for escalating asthma treatment using different preventer inhalers (which contain steroids) or other medicines. The vast majority of asthma can be well controlled as long as medicines are taken regularly and correctly. If things are not going well, your practice nurse or doctor will need to check you are using the inhalers correctly and to ensure that your child is taking them regularly. They should also ask about symptoms of rhinitis (see Chapter 10) as this is an important cause of poor asthma control and is why many asthma attacks occur in the pollen season. Remember that when symptoms improve with regular asthma medicines, you need to keep taking them. Asthma is still a major killer in the UK and must be taken seriously.

Emergency plan

If your child is diagnosed with asthma, the emergency plan for an allergic reaction must be changed to include giving their inhalers (see pages 92 and 261). Up to 10 puffs of the reliever should be given via a spacer device to try to prevent the allergic reaction changing from a mild to a severe one involving the breathing system. Any child with food allergy and asthma should also be prescribed and trained how to use adrenaline autoinjectors (see page 118). If your asthmatic child has an allergic reaction, it is often worth considering giving a single dose of oral steroid medicine to stop the asthma flaring up a few hours later. This should be on your emergency treatment plan.

Outgrowing Asthma

Most children with mild, intermittent asthma will outgrow their asthma completely or have mild asthma in adulthood. More severe childhood asthma or atopic symptoms increase the risk of asthma persisting or returning in adulthood. In addition to this, exposing your child to passive cigarette smoke or smoking decreases the likelihood of outgrowing asthma. Early intervention with anti-inflammatory therapy, such as appropriate use of oral corticosteroids, may prevent the progression of the disease and result in improved lung performance in later life.

CHAPTER 12
Advances in Managing Food Allergy

Allergic disease – the umbrella term that covers food allergy, eczema, asthma and allergic rhinitis – is understood more now than in the past. As we have previously discussed, what happens in the body during an allergic reaction is also better recognised – at least for immediate, IgE mediated reactions. Why it happens, and how exactly to prevent it or cure it is, unfortunately, less well understood. However, research is taking place all the time and the study of allergies is receiving much attention because of the huge increase in the number of sufferers that have been seen over the past decades.

This focus on research into allergies has meant that new strategies to change how the body responds during an allergic reaction and new methods of treatment are being trialled. There are now promising forms of treatment, called immunotherapy, which are in their infancy but could possibly be the future of allergy treatment. This chapter will briefly discuss these developments and touch on the current research within the field of allergy in order to show the bigger picture of managing your child's symptoms. Chapter 7 discusses some everyday ways to manage your child's allergies.

Food Elimination

The central pillar of food allergy management is avoidance of the offending allergen. In the case of milk allergy, especially as it is often the main source of nutrition in the child, avoidance affects everything. The involvement of a paediatric dietician is key. Education on how to read food labels and avoid milk as well as choosing an appropriate substitute that ensures complete nutrition requires considerable expertise. Further education on how to recognise and treat the reactions that may result from accidental exposure is also important. Regular follow-up to monitor growth and the possible development of tolerance is also needed, as is a holistic approach to ensure the early recognition and treatment of the other emerging allergic conditions that your child may have.

As I was breastfeeding S, they suggested that I came off dairy for a week and see what happened to his symptoms. Within two days he turned into a very content, smiley little baby who rarely cried, the difference was astonishing.

HANNAH, MUM OF S

I took milk out of my diet and the eczema significantly improved. This was sometime around Christmas 2009 – nine months since it first appeared, and so months of agony for the poor boys, very little sleep for any of us and a broken mummy.

EMMA, MUM OF CAMERON AND DILLON

Food elimination is a challenge of its own but has huge rewards for your child and little detriment, if carried out carefully and managed well.

Is Complete Avoidance the Answer?

Recent research has established that up to 70 per cent of children with IgE mediated milk and egg allergy are able to tolerate baked milk or egg in their diet. This can make life much easier. Such children tend to have a milder type of milk or egg allergy associated with milder reactions, smaller allergy tests and early outgrowing. New studies suggest that introducing baked egg or milk to the diet when it can be tolerated may also speed up the process of outgrowing the whole milk or egg allergy. However, testing to differentiate children who are and are not tolerant to baked milk or egg is limited and children can have severe reactions. This means that supervised challenge testing, best directed by a specialist doctor, is required. You should discuss this with your doctor if you think it may be relevant.

Modifying the Immune System – Desensitisation

Immunotherapy works by modifying the way that the body reacts to an allergenic substance, in order to desensitise the allergy sufferer. The term 'desensitise' means that the immune system is less sensitive and less likely to react to the allergen and that only greater levels of exposure will cause a reaction. Unfortunately, this type of approach has only proved useful for IgE but not non-IgE mediated reactions. If you remember back to Chapter 1, we looked at how the body reacts incorrectly to food because the immune system wrongly recognises harmless food proteins such as egg protein, identifying them as harmful. This causes the immune system to react, resulting in an allergic response with the itching, swelling and other symptoms that you see in your child.

By changing the body's immune system, scientists believe that they can change the way that the body reacts to a harmless food protein and therefore change the immune response and ultimately reduce any allergic response. This is the principle behind desensitisation. It is now recognised as a highly specific and effective method to treat certain types of allergy. The concept is not new. Immunotherapy has been in use for over a hundred years in the treatment of allergic rhinitis to grass pollen. It is also well established in the management of bee and wasp venom allergy.

Desensitisation and pollen allergy

To desensitise the allergic rhinitis sufferer, drops or tablets of the pollen allergen are placed under the tongue of the sufferer in increasing doses. This can also be done with injections. As a result, the allergic rhinitis sufferer becomes desensitised to pollen over time, with the effect increasing over the course of a three-year period of desensitisation. Occasionally, this can lead to an almost complete resolution in symptoms but more often it simply reduces them to more manageable levels. After a three-year period of treatment the effect usually persists even though the treatment has been stopped. Desensitisation with pollen has also been shown, within this group of allergic rhinitis sufferers, to reduce the risk of progression of allergic disease from allergic rhinitis to asthma, which is something that is otherwise very common. While the mechanism by which desensitisation works remains unclear, it is starting to unravel. The clear success of desensitisation in allergic rhinitis sufferers has led to researchers and clinicians who specialise in allergy to look at similar methods of treatment for other allergies, including food allergy.

Desensitisation and food allergy

Desensitisation with food allergy involves the administration of the food allergen to the patient in small but increasing doses. Most trials give the child a very small amount of the allergen to eat or drink with close observation and then keep the tolerated level in the diet at home on a regular basis. The aim is to raise the level of allergen your child can ingest and cope with, without having a reaction. Once this is achieved, a maintenance dose is continued to uphold this desensitisation.

Unfortunately, there have been two troubling issues with this treatment. The first is the sometimes severe side-effects, which have led to attempts at injection desensitisation to food being abandoned. There are also issues with desensitization by placing the allergen in the mouth, which can cause occasional but severe reactions. Another issue is the lack of long-lasting effects seen once consumption of the allergen is stopped in many children. Desensitisation with food seems to have a temporary effect, lasting only for the duration of active treatment. In other words, the child does not develop tolerance (the ability to ingest the allergen without symptoms despite periods of allergen avoidance). After a period of avoiding the allergenic food, your child will react again to the allergenic food when it is ingested. Is it worth the effort and risk of ingesting regular doses when the end result is still not being rid of the allergy? Desensitisation for food allergy is also not in everyday use in the clinical setting as yet but remains the subject of intense study.

Current Studies

Ongoing research into the prevention of anaphylaxis and food allergy in general is vital. New and novel therapeutic approaches with the aim of reducing reaction, encouraging tolerance or curing food allergy are emerging as knowledge is advancing. Immunotherapy is taking an increasingly important role. Remarkable progress has been made within the field of food allergy treatment. As these strategies progress beyond the research stage, disease-modifying therapies rather than food avoidance may become the standard of care, and the increasing incidence of anaphylaxis occurring may even be reversed over the next decade.

There are studies that have been carried out and are ongoing which look at immunotherapy for peanut, milk and egg allergies. Further studies are needed, however, and there are risks involved. A number of children drop out of the studies because of allergic reactions and gastro-intestinal symptoms. The studies are looking at the use of different ways to administer the food allergen, as well as measuring the effect that it is having on the child. The methods being used are oral immunotherapy, where the allergen is ingested, which we have discussed. There is also sublingual immunotherapy, which involves placing a few drops of the allergen under the tongue, as is used with the pollen allergy desensitisation. With food allergy, it has been found to induce desensitisation but not as effectively as oral treatment or ingestion. The third method is called epicutaneous immunotherapy, where the allergen is given via a skin patch. This is being trialled with milk allergy sufferers and there is currently a peanut trial underway. Finally, there is immunotherapy with modified food proteins, which has been shown to reduce side-effects of allergen exposure.

It is still early days for food immunotherapy and much more research is needed. Immunotherapy to induce desensitisation to food is not used routinely in allergy clinics in the NHS. However, results from trials are promising and it is an area that is likely to be in mainstream use in the future, especially for those who are unlikely to become tolerant to a food naturally, such as those with peanut allergy.

Anti-IgE therapy

There may be a role for anti-IgE therapies in treating food allergy. In Chapter 1 we discussed IgE, the antibody that identifies the harmless food protein and thereby triggers the immune response. IgE also plays a pivotal role in severe and anaphylactic food-related reactions. Therefore, treating the allergy sufferer with an injection therapy to block the actions of IgE is a promising idea.

One study using this method has shown that peanut allergy sufferers treated with anti-IgE therapy react only to a much higher level of peanut protein, meaning that they tolerate greater levels of peanut (see References, page 281). Astonishingly, the level that the sufferer can then tolerate may be much higher than the level that caused anaphylaxis through accidental exposure. While these results are encouraging in terms of the prevention of anaphylaxis, the method only works if the sufferer has regular injections, which are very expensive. Research now is therefore looking at combining anti-IgE therapy with desensitisation (see page 157). It is hoped that this combination may reduce the amount of side-effects and nasty reactions that the sufferer experiences while going through the process of desensitisation, but that once desensitised the regular injections can be stopped.

Early diet changes

There is other research looking at changing a child's diet early in life. The aim is to promote the development of tolerance as a way of avoiding allergy developing in children who may be prone to it. One promising example is the LEAP study (www.leapstudy.co.uk), which has taken children aged 4–10 months who have eczema and/or egg allergy. These children carry a 20 per cent risk of developing peanut allergy. The children were randomly split into two groups, one given peanut protein as a weaning food and one told to avoid it. The study is ongoing, but results when the children are five will be compared. It is hoped that the children in the group that have been exposed early to peanut protein will have less incidences of peanut allergy.

Chinese herbal medicine

Another exciting line of investigation in the treatment of food allergy is the use of Chinese herbs. Animal trials have found that treatment of food allergies with Chinese herbs is safe, straightforward and well tolerated. However, while animal trials have shown good results, human trials are in their early stages. Again, much more research is needed before this could be a successful way to treat food allergy.

CHAPTER 13
Preventing Food Allergies

The greatest incidence of food allergy is in the first few years of life, affecting 5–15 per cent of children in the first year, if you include both IgE and non-IgE mediated allergies (see Chapters 1 and 2). Children are most likely to have IgE mediated allergies to cow's milk and eggs, as well as nuts, fish and shellfish, while non-IgE mediated reactions are most commonly to milk and soy. This chapter discusses theories behind allergy development and ways to prevent allergies from developing in high-risk families. While this is not helpful if you already have an allergic child, it is worth discussing within the context of any future children you may be planning.

Essentials

- There remains no clear way to prevent food allergies in high-risk children.
- The best recommendation for families at high risk of allergic disease is breastfeeding for the first 4–6 months exclusively and not smoking.
- Introduction of solid foods, even allergenic ones, need not be delayed beyond 4–6 months.

Protective Influences against Food Allergy in Pregnancy

There are some steps you can take during pregnancy to reduce the risk of your child developing allergies.

Vitamin D

Our paediatrician told us that the best way to prevent allergy in another child would be to conceive in a hot, sunny climate. I asked for that in writing! He seems to have a point, however. There is some evidence to show high maternal vitamin D intake during pregnancy is associated with a lower risk of asthma in preschool children. This, plus the fact that vitamin D in the lab can improve the immune response, makes vitamin D the target of clinical trials at the moment. Currently, however, there is yet to be any evidence that taking a vitamin D supplement reduces risk.

Probiotics

The studies looking at maternal probiotic and child supplements have had varying results with the overall recommendation that probiotics, especially if introduced prenatally, do have the potential to prevent or lower the incidence of eczema in children. More research is needed especially as any effect may relate to what species of bacteria are used and the dose. It is therefore incredibly hard to guess what may or may not be helpful.

Fish oils

Studies looking at increased levels of fish oils in the diet have been inconclusive. It is advised that pregnant women do not eat more than two portions of oily fish per week, however, and if you do decide to take a fish oil supplement, take one that does not contain vitamin A as this has been shown to be potentially harmful to the unborn child.

The mother's diet

Although it seems plausible, it does not seem to be the case that allergies develop in the unborn child during pregnancy. One British study looked at the blood tests taken at birth of children who later turned out to have peanut allergy – none of them had any allergic antibody to peanuts detectable in those first blood samples. An American study found no difference in food allergy among children whose mothers avoided allergenic foods in pregnancy when compared to those who didn't. It is therefore now widely accepted that avoidance diets during pregnancy should not be recommended as a way to prevent allergenic disease. For every pregnant woman, the most important advice is to eat a healthy, balanced diet.

The UK Government's advice about peanut consumption during pregnancy and breastfeeding has changed in recent years. The advice now is that pregnant women and breastfeeding mothers can eat peanuts or food containing peanuts, regardless of whether there is a family history of peanut allergy (www.food.gov.uk). Maternal consumption of peanut or any other common allergen during these periods simply doesn't seem to make a difference either way to the risk of food allergies in the child.

Fruit and vegetable intake is important during pregnancy and again there are some studies linking insufficient fruit intake with asthma up to the age of two years. There are also studies linking low levels of vitamin E in the mother's diet with asthma development in the under-fives. However, none of this is conclusive and there are no guidelines as yet.

Smoking

Smoking when pregnant has many harmful effects to the unborn child, with a particular link to the development of asthma, which would further compromise a child who then went on to develop allergies.

Protective Influences against Food Allergy in Postnatal Women

Once your baby is born, there are further measures you can take to reduce the risk of him developing allergies.

Breastfeeding

Breastfeeding exclusively for four or more months from birth is associated with a reduced risk of your child developing eczema and asthma. Breast milk has a complex nature and the food allergens that are passed to the child from the mother may in fact allow your baby to get used to them without reaction. Therefore, a period of exclusive breastfeeding is recommended.

Breastfeeding is widely recommended for the nutritional, immunological and psychological benefits to the child. However, studies have found milk, egg, peanut and wheat allergens in breast milk two to six hours after the mother has eaten them. The risk, therefore, is that these allergens are passed in the breast milk to the child and sensitisation occurs. However, there is very good evidence from well-conducted studies that the mother's diet during breastfeeding has no impact on the likelihood of food allergy developing. As a result, all of the international guidelines are clear that there is no value in avoiding specific foods during breastfeeding. The fact that some foods get through to the breast milk does mean that once your child has developed a food allergy, the food in mum's diet can lead to symptoms. The allergen can remain in the breast milk for 1–4 days.

I became aware of this during one long breastfeeding session. Minutes into every feed, Zach's cheeks, neck and ears would become raised, develop red streaks and he would begin itching. His face would become red and his lips swollen, and a rash would appear on his arms and legs. This was often accompanied by what looked like stomach ache and constipation for some time after the end of the feed. This was when I started to investigate cow's milk protein allergy and I now realise that this was the result of him reacting to milk in my own diet via the breast milk. So, food in the mum's diet can cause symptoms in the allergic child. However, having these foods during breastfeeding isn't the cause of those allergies, so there is no value cutting anything out unless your child is getting symptoms.

Despite the presence of allergens, exclusive breastfeeding for at least four months is recommended to reduce the risk of eczema in infancy, especially in high-risk families. Of course, breastfeeding has lots of other health benefits. As well as encouraging better bonding… it's free. Studies in Europe have also shown that if you can't exclusively breastfeed for the first four months, then using a broken-down formula (partially or extensively hydrolysed casein-based formula) may decrease the risks of developing eczema for the subsequent 10 years, especially if there is a history of eczema in the mother. If you can't exclusively breastfeed for four months, then discuss this with your GP who may be happy to prescribe an appropriate formula to reduce the risks to your baby.

The hygiene hypothesis

This 'clean child theory' is the most common theory as to why there has been an increase in allergies. Reduced exposure to dirt and infection in childhood has led to a rise in eczema and asthma as our immune systems are not maturing quickly. There is evidence that exposure to bacteria stimulates and shapes early immune development. Research has shown that owning a pet, growing up on a farm or unhygienic contact with older siblings are all associated with protection from certain allergies and therefore a lower occurrence of allergies, possibly due to increased bacterial exposure. However, there is no good evidence to show that having a dirty household protects from allergy and certainly no evidence that avoiding vaccination reduces the risk either. Vaccination is still recommended in all children.

Formula milk

There is no evidence that the use of soy formula is effective at preventing food allergy or intolerance in high-risk groups. It is a safe alternative, however, to cow's milk formula in the majority of children with cow's milk allergy after screening to rule out co-existing soy allergy but not recommended until after six months due to the high levels of plant oestrogens.

Weaning

There is no clear evidence that the delayed introduction of foods beyond 4–6 months helps prevent the development of allergies. However, there is increasing interest in the role of early introduction of certain allergens into the child's diet as a way of reducing the risk of food allergy. This is based on evidence that in some countries, where peanut is used as a weaning food, levels of peanut allergy are very low, even among high-risk children. There are large studies underway to investigate this so for the moment the advice is still to aim to exclusively breastfeed for 4–6 months, that introducing first additional foods is safe from 17 weeks and that delaying the introduction of allergenic foods (as was advised in previous years) is of no benefit.

CHAPTER 14
Weaning and Nutrition

Weaning should be an exciting developmental milestone. It is a time when your child begins to show likes and dislikes, reacting to tastes and flavours and taking on the challenges of managing different textures. The timing of weaning can unfortunately come during the process of diagnosis of food allergy, making it even more confusing. As a parent, not only do you need to get to grips with weaning, but you need to get to grips with what allergies are and what they look like – which foods are safe for your child and which are not and, above all, you need to do it fast. That is a challenge. Weaning is one of the hardest journeys that you take as the parent or carer of a child with food allergies. You may have started to discuss your concerns with friends, family and even your GP, but whether your child has a formal diagnosis of food allergy or not, every day you have the challenge of introducing new foods and flavours into your child's diet. However, with careful planning and an informed approach, it is possible to wean your baby successfully.

My youngest, Harry was diagnosed at six months old with a milk and egg allergy. After exclusively breastfeeding, I absentmindedly tried him with some porridge containing skimmed milk powder and he vomited and came up in hives. Due to his age and not knowing if I could give antihistamines, I called 999. He was referred immediately and seen by the allergy clinic a month later where they tested for these allergies and the ones Sam [his older brother] has too. Only the milk and egg were positive. I carried on breastfeeding until 10½ months and during this time his sleep was dreadful. I now wonder if he wasn't tolerating the dairy coming through my milk. I stopped breastfeeding and he went on to a hypoallergenic formula, which suits him well and he now sleeps much better.

KATHRYN, MUM OF SAM AND HARRY

Weaning... a Journey into the Unknown

If your child has food allergies, weaning can become a frightening time for you as a parent, especially if you have already experienced your child having a food-related reaction. You may suspect that your child has allergies but not be sure to which foods or to what extent she is allergic.

The weaning process was a bit hit and miss with Sam as we had no experience of food allergies or weaning! I hated it, never knowing whether or not he would have a reaction to food. It was a very stressful time. With Harry [second child], I was very slow, cautious and meticulous. I waited... between each new food and recorded it in a diary. I was still very nervous but felt a bit more prepared.

KATHRYN, MUM OF SAM AND HARRY

Food is an integral part of social gatherings. Without planning and care, not only the child who is allergic but also the family is at risk of exclusion. Eating competence is also vitally important to the socialisation of a child. Children with food allergies are at risk of developing food aversions and self-limited diets, beyond the elimination diet. Children as well as their parents can become anxious about food. Zach, at three-and-a-half, recently told me that he worries when he eats food. While that was awful to hear, I do understand and just have to work harder to give him more confidence in the food he is given to eat.

The usual baby books that other parents are following no longer fully apply to your situation, or can only be used in part. They offer great recipe ideas that you can use with substitute ingredients, as well as guides on progression of foods and textures, but otherwise can be limited. So what should you do? Without following all the new foods that are recommended, how do you ensure your baby has a wide experience of flavours and textures and how do you ensure that nutritionally she has the best start in life?

Above all, how do you keep your baby safe and free from allergic reaction? And how do you keep the anxiety at bay and still allow weaning to be exciting and experimental?

This chapter and chapters 15 and 16 aim to tackle these questions, providing ideas, recipes and suggestions that will give you some of the control back, answer your questions, take away some worry and allow you to focus on your child.

Essentials

Advice from a dietician is essential if you are going to cut foods out of your child's diet. The NICE guidelines on food allergy are very clear that any child with food allergies should have the opportunity to consult a dietician – make sure you get this specialist help.

- Milk is the most important food in the first year.
- Substitute mammalian milk such as sheep or goat is never suitable for children aged under 12 months.
- Rice-based milk is not recommended for children under the age of four-and-a-half years.

- Soy-based infant formula can be used in children from six months, where appropriate.
- Fortified soya, oat, coconut, almond, hazelnut, pea or quinoa milk can be used for cooking but are not suitable as a main drink in the under-twos.
- Extensively hydrolysed or amino acid infant formula for milk allergy needs to be prescribed by a GP.
- Offer a varied diet with adequate nutritional substitutes.
- There is currently no evidence that delaying the introduction of solid food beyond 4–6 months of age has a significant protective effect on the development of atopic disease.
- Use the three-day wait rule only for high-risk foods likely to cause delayed allergy (milk, egg, soy, wheat) when weaning.
- Use a food reaction diary to remember and record progress and reactions.
- Make a safe food checklist as you wean.

The Dietician

The key to successful weaning on to solids with a child with food allergies is to manage the symptoms, strictly avoid the food allergens yet, with the help of a dietician and nutritional advice, ensure an ongoing well-balanced diet. Easy!

When S was four months I asked for a referral to a dietician and we were seen when he was five months – finally I felt we were in safe hands. She listened to S's history, his symptoms, his reactions and helped us start him on a hypoallergenic formula to go alongside my breast milk as I had decided to start weaning him on to formula. Our dietician has continued to review S every six months and has been a good support.

HANNAH, MUM OF S

As the saying goes 'breast is best'. It is the best for your baby's immune system and has been shown to have a long-lasting impact on health and disease. The World Health Organization and the Department of Health (2003) recommend that all babies should be exclusively breastfed for the first six months and then solids introduced at six months. However, some babies can have food allergies through breast milk and so some mothers face a difficult dilemma.

It is known that food proteins pass through breast milk and can cause allergic reactions, particularly milk, soy and egg. In this situation, it is best to seek advice from your GP, allergist or dietician before you either eliminate the suspect foods from your diet and continue breastfeeding (usually the preferred option), or stop breastfeeding all together and try a hypoallergenic (extensively hydrolysed or amino acid) formula.

This decision is entirely personal. If you decide to stop breastfeeding, take it slowly as it can be an emotional time and you need to reduce your milk supply slowly and ensure your child is getting enough formula milk.

This chapter is subjective and discusses other parents' stories and experiences. We do not recommend that you eliminate foods from your diet if breastfeeding and we recommend that you seek only professional dietetic support for your child. *It is vital that your child is seen by a qualified, specialist dietician.* The aim is to show you that, while this stage can be a huge challenge, it doesn't have to be frightening.

Nutrition

••

Great care must be taken to provide adequate nutrition for the growth and development of every child. If your child has reacted to a food, you will naturally have stopped giving your child that food until you are given medical guidance. This is the right and proper thing to do. However, it is vital that you seek medical help, firstly from your GP and then through referral to a dietician and allergy specialist.

> *I worry that Felix has a limited diet, that he is affected nutritionally and that his health will be affected because of it.*

EMILY, MUM OF FELIX

If your child has had food removed from her diet, because of suspected food allergies, more attention is needed to provide the nutrient-rich food she requires. Children with food allergies are at risk of inadequate nutritional intake, mainly due to inadequate replacement of nutrients, which are in the eliminated foods.

What happens when a food group is removed?

The main food groups include fruit and vegetables, carbohydrates, protein, dairy and dietary fat. These groups provide vitamins, minerals, fibre and calories. Below is a summary of the nutritional elements of the most common food groups eliminated because of allergy and suggested ways to replace these to help ensure that your child has a balanced, nutritionally adequate diet. This list is by no means complete and, again, please liaise with a qualified dietician for further nutritional advice.

Our experience

I had to go to the GP on numerous occasions to discuss my suspicions about Zach's allergies to something in my breast milk. It appeared that I was not being listened to, however, so I decided to get some evidence together and provide proof by eliminating cow's milk from my diet for two weeks to note any changes in Zach. His symptoms did improve initially but then deteriorated again. By this point, Zach was nearly four months old and we were exhausted and decided to try some baby formula for hungry babies, following up the helpful suggestion that maybe his crying and poor sleep were due to hunger. We thought that, despite Zach's eczema, being hungry was worse than itching. I was also wondering if my breast milk was insufficient to sustain his appetite. My husband therefore gave Zach a bottle of formula before bed. Within minutes we had proof of his allergies and level of suffering. His face became bright red, his eyelids and lips swelled and he began to cry. Next, he was sick and had diarrhoea. We didn't call an ambulance, but had I been alone, I would have done. Eventually he stopped crying and fell asleep snoring. The silver lining to that horrendous night was that finally we had the proof we needed to get the GPs to listen. The next day I relayed the events and thankfully a referral was made to a community paediatrician. The same GP also provided stronger steroids and a thick moisturiser to start a skincare regime for Zach. It is unacceptable that my concerns were not listened to until Zach's reaction was made crystal clear by giving him baby formula. However, that evidence was all we needed to begin to put an end to Zach's suffering and the heartache that we had been going through.

We had to wait a couple of months for Zach to see the paediatrician. I was still breastfeeding and had eliminated milk and soy from my diet, at the suggestion of the health visitor that dairy and soy allergies often come hand in hand. I was desperate for a coffee with proper milk, especially as at eight months old Zach was still waking every two hours days and night for a feed. The health visitors in the meantime had referred us to a dietician. I had so many questions and I needed some answers, because at five months, we began to wean Zach on to puréed foods. I needed to know which milk I could use for the baby rice. I also wanted to know about a formula that Zach could be given and whether I could wean him using rice milk or oat milk.

I had felt quite excited about the weaning process, loving the thought of Zach trying flavours, textures and watching his reaction. However, for me, the whole process became filled with anxiety. As I followed the baby weaning plans of fruit, vegetable, rice, it became clear that Zach had multiple allergies. While eating food such as avocado, mango and lentils, he would have what I now know are oral reactions – he looked like he had waxed his top lip or his cheek rash would appear. He also had delayed reactions to the daytime foods that he had eaten where he would develop dermatitis over his whole body or he would be constipated and very unsettled. I decided not to progress to the allergenic foods, such as eggs, cheese and yoghurt (as they contain milk protein), and thank goodness I didn't as he would have had a severe reaction. I basically needed more information than that which I was working out for myself from weaning books. I needed to know about food groups, allergenic foods, which to avoid and I needed some direction but there was none available to me. The whole time I was terrified that with one mouthful, I would endanger Zach's life. It sounds dramatic, but the unknown is so frightening. Another constant anxiety of mine while weaning Zach was his nutrition. I had no idea what was in the foods that I was eliminating from his diet. I therefore had no idea how to replace these nutrients. He had vitamin drops but I think that his nutrition could have been improved. If I'd have been able to get more advice from a dietician, I would have felt more confident in the process of eliminating food. It is important not to do guesswork when it comes to food elimination but to seek the advice of a specialist dietician who has the tools to help and guide you.

Cow's Milk Protein Allergy

A diet free from cow's milk eliminates cow's milk proteins (casein and whey) and milk sugar (lactose). The nutritional effect of cow's milk elimination can be great because milk is often the primary source of fat, protein, calcium and vitamins and it is the main food for a child. Finding a nutritionally dense substitute is essential. If you can achieve this early on in your child's diagnosis, a lot of the anxiety about allergies and the nutritional consequences that food elimination can have will be removed.

It is worth remembering that if you are breastfeeding your child and you are on a cow's milk protein elimination diet, the nutritional implications are huge for you as well. As the mother, your diet needs to be assessed for your own health and for the composition of the breast milk that you are producing. A calcium supplement and may be recommended. Again, a dietician can do this via a referral from your GP.

Milk substitute formulas

For the first year of life, breast milk or formula is given to children without cow's milk protein allergy because ordinary cow's, sheep's or goat's milk does not provide adequate iron and other nutrients. Cow's milk can be used in cooking or mixed with cereals for weaning after six months, but not as a main drink. After one year of age, children can be moved from breast milk or formula to cow's milk. The first thing you need to know when your child has a suspected or confirmed cow's milk protein allergy is that child formula milk is made from cow's milk. This means that it is not suitable for your child.

Cow's milk substitute formulas:

- Extensively hydrolysed formulas and amino acid based formulas must be prescribed by a GP.
- Partially hydrolysed formulas are available but are not suitable for milk allergy.
- Soya-based formula is not recommended for babies under the age of 6 months.

Alternative milks

- Non-formula fortified alternative milks such as almond or oat will not provide adequate nutrients in infancy.
- Rice milk is not recommended in children under four and a half years old.
- Sheep's or goat's milk is not recommended for cow's milk allergy as the proteins are very similar and will most likely cause reactions.

Cow's milk formula alternatives

For formula-fed children or for those weaning off breast milk, there are different types of formula available. These include extensively hydrolysed formula, amino acid formula and soya formula. The British Dietetic Association Paediatric Group do not recommend soya formulas for children under the age of six months due to levels of phytoestrogens and the common cross reactivity with cow's milk protein allergy.

The majority of children with cow's milk protein allergy tolerate extensively hydrolysed formulas. Hydrolysis is the process by which proteins from milk are broken down to make it less allergenic – a variety of extensively and partially hydrolysed alternatives to dairy-based formula are available. Partially hydrolysed formulas are not suitable for a child with cow's milk protein allergy. If your child still shows some allergic symptoms, or she does not have a complete resolution of her symptoms when drinking extensively hydrolysed formulas, an amino acid formula may be used. Amino acid-based formulas are fully synthetic formulas, which are essentially invisible to the immune system. Therefore, there is no risk at all to children with cow's milk protein allergy. In some children with severe reactions to milk, or when they are clearly already reacting to cow's milk through maternal breast milk (and are thus very sensitive), the doctors may suggest going straight on to an amino acid formula. Extensively hydrolysed and amino acid formulas are very expensive but are available on prescription.

The British Dietetic Association state that hypoallergenic formulas have a different smell and taste, which most babies under six months will accept. For those who are older and for children who have delayed, non-IgE mediated allergic reactions, it is helpful to gradually introduce the new milk by mixing it with their usual milk. When you change your baby's formula, it is worth knowing that hypoallergenic formula can make your child's poo dark green and she may need to open her bowels less often. This is nothing to worry about. There are different formulas for different ages and your dietician will be able to advise you as to which is most appropriate for your child.

Alternative milks

The non-formula alternative milks will not provide adequate nutrients during infancy. For example, milks such as almond milk are enriched to provide adequate calcium and vitamin D, but have little protein and are low in fat. Enriched oat milk contains about half the protein of cow's milk. These milks may have a place over the age of one. Rice milk is not recommended under four and a half years of age.

Milk-allergic babies

Breast milk, or fortified infant formula, must still remain the mainstay of your baby's diet as it contains all of the nutrients that she needs. Once your allergic baby is weaned, most need up to 600 ml (20 fl oz) of hypoallergenic formula a day to meet their nutritional requirements. If your baby consumes less, let your dietician know as a supplement may be needed. Children over one year generally need 300 ml (10 fl oz) of milk substitute each day. If you are concerned that your child is not drinking this much, try to add milk to her diet through breakfast cereal and in cooking. Again, your child's dietician can check the nutritional content of the rest of your baby's diet and adjust the requirements needed.

The Department of Health recommends giving a supplement of vitamin D and A to all children over six months who are being given breast milk as their main milk source, those at risk of vitamin D deficiency, any child under one who is not consuming 600 ml (20 fl oz) or above of child formula a day and for all 1–5-year-olds.

> *I continued my dairy-free diet and fed S until he was six months, then we weaned him on to a prescribed hypoallergenic formula, which he loves!*
>
> HANNAH, MUM OF S

For cooking, your baby's prescribed formula milk can be used and many milk manufacturers provide recipes and lots of other information about allergies on their websites (see page 258). It is also feasible to use oat or soya milk, once your child is older than 12 months. These milks are available from the supermarket, come in fresh and long life but make sure you use the ones fortified with calcium and vitamins.

Tip: Ask the doctor to write out a prescription for multiple tins of your prescription milk. You will find that you go through a lot of it. Always have a back-up alternative milk in the cupboard for those times when you may run out of milk.

> *Since S's diagnosis I experienced a stroppy GP who asked how long his practice would have to pay for his formula, implying that my son's allergy was a financial drain on his practice. I promptly found a new practice.*
>
> HANNAH, MUM OF S

Wheat Allergy

To eliminate wheat from your child's diet, many food products such as bread, pasta, cereals, crackers, cookies and cakes must be avoided. Wheat is also often used as a minor ingredient in foods such as condiments, soups, soy sauce and jellybeans. Gluten-free products and 'very low gluten' products may still contain other proteins found in wheat (albumins, globulins and starch granule proteins), so these might not be suitable. Wheat provides carbohydrates, thiamin, niacin, riboflavin, iron, folic acid and fibre. Wheat is also found in Play-Doh.

There are many alternative flours available such as rice, corn, quinoa, gram and millet, which may be suitable. Elimination of wheat products has a significant nutritional impact, particularly for vitamin B and fibre. Vitamin B can be replaced using the foods mentioned above and fibre through alternative grains. Fruit and vegetables are also high in fibre.

Egg Allergy

Egg contributes protein, vitamin B12, riboflavin, pantothenic acid, biotin and selenium to the diet. Many foods supply these nutrients and therefore your child's diet will not generally be compromised if egg allergy stands alone.

Egg is, however, a common ingredient in many foods such as meatballs, baked goods and casseroles. Home-cooking of these foods using an egg replacement will enable these foods to be eaten. Some versions of these foods that are free from egg are also available. There are ingredients such as applesauce, banana or flaxseed that can be used to replace egg in cooking (see page 201). Some commercially available egg replacers designed for home baking do, however, contain egg protein and are therefore not suitable.

Soybean Allergy

Soybean protein is in a variety of ingredients, yet many allergy sufferers can tolerate soy oil or soy lecithin. Again, please seek the advice of your child's dietician. Soy is nutritionally dense and provides protein but the nutrients lost due to its elimination are easily replaced. It is not usually, however, a major component in a child's diet but may have a link to cow's milk protein allergy.

Peanut Allergy

Avoidance of peanut and other tree nuts in a diet does not pose any threat to nutrition.

Note: Please see the Resources section on pages 256–8 for information about where to buy 'free from' foods and Chapter 16 for some 'free from' recipes, which cover the many social and celebratory events in life.

When to Wean

Begin weaning at around six months of age and not before your baby is 17 weeks old. From the food allergy point of view there have been conflicting reports about when to introduce solids. However, currently it appears that there is no definite evidence either way in terms of when to start weaning to avoid developing further allergies. There is good evidence that there is no value in delaying the introduction of allergenic foods though. Therefore, follow the normal guidelines of your baby's age, physical development and signs of hunger and interest in other food.

How to start

Ideally your dietician or paediatrician will be on hand and able to guide you through this process. Please do always seek professional medical advice before trying any of the major allergenic foods with your child. It is also not safe to eliminate a food from your baby's diet unless you are sure that it needs to be eliminated, again having sought medical advice. Unnecessary elimination could lead to poor nutrition, while giving an allergenic food could result in a dangerous life-threatening reaction for your child.

Food diary

It is essential to seek advice from a dietician and helpful to keep a food diary. The dietician can then look through your child's food diary and analyse her diet over a period of two weeks, calculating the levels of calcium, protein and other nutrients. Keep a diary of milk and food intake over the course of two weeks including one weekend. While you are waiting to see a dietician, you can complete the food diary. This way you have a headstart when meeting with the dietician for the first time.

Include in the diary the brands of foods, such as cheese and yoghurts, that your child is eating as each has different nutritional levels that can be specifically calculated. The dietician will then be able to advise you about which milk to use as a drink and in cooking and which brands of alternative foods to buy to maximise the nutritional benefits. Calcium syrup supplement is usually available for children, as are vitamin drops. Both are available on prescription and are well worth considering in discussion with your GP while waiting to be seen by a dietician.

When we saw the dietician for the first time with Zach, she calculated his calcium intake on an estimation of the Neocate formula he was drinking. The dietician also advised a calcium syrup supplement, soy yoghurt, custards and cheese, which we could then add to Zach's diet. I finally felt equipped to manage my son's allergies. I knew which foods to avoid, had vitamin drops and calcium supplements, and was using some soy food replacements.

	Milk	Breakfast	Snack	Lunch	Snack	Dinner	Milk
Day 1							
Day 2							
Day 3							
Day 4							
Day 5							
Day 6							
Day 7							
Day 8							
Day 9							
Day 10							
Day 11							
Day 12							
Day 13							
Day 14							

I managed weaning with guidance from our dietician and a lot of online research! Annabel Karmel's book (a commonly used weaning book) was useful. I also introduced new (allergenic) foods very slowly... As S's reactions were always delayed, this did present a few challenges as I wasn't always sure what was causing his symptoms. This is a process we are still going through and he is now 16 months old.

HANNAH, MUM OF S

Where to start

In order to wean safely, it is best to take it slowly. Begin weaning with low-allergenic foods such as puréed rice, potatoes, and vegetables mixed with a little of your baby's usual milk. It is important to know the high- and low-risk foods and only try the low-risk ones, without supervision. There are still uncertainties about the best time to introduce more allergenic foods. Take advice from a dietician or allergist before trying any high-risk foods and introduce only one at a time. It is also useful to make a list of safe foods, which you can add to as time goes on. That way you can learn and remember easily and compile your own checklist of safe ingredients, which could act as a prompt for you when food shopping (see Chapter 7).

I remember when Zach was about nine months old, one of my friends was giving her baby, who was the same age as Zach, a lamb hotpot purée, while I was still stuck on carrot and parsnip purée! You just have to learn to adapt and not compare yourself or your baby with others.

For weaning my advice would be to ignore what other mothers are doing. I remember being alarmed at the variety of foods other babies were eating when S was gradually expanding his diet. It's so important to give them time during weaning so try not to feel under pressure to hurry it.

HANNAH, MUM OF S

Common Allergenic Foods

In IgE mediated allergy, most significant allergic reactions to foods are due to milk, egg, peanuts, tree nuts, fish, shellfish, wheat, sesame and soy. These foods are the major food allergens so a greater degree of caution is warranted for the introduction of these foods. However, previous advice to delay the introduction of allergenic foods has not proven to be helpful in reducing the risk of food allergy and is not advisable. If there is a known food allergy then discuss the introduction of other allergenic foods with your doctor or dietician but do not fall into the trap of putting this off. They may recommend allergy testing to get the required reassurance to confidently introduce the food.

Weaning and Reactions

Only a limited number of foods typically lead to a delayed allergic reaction. These are milk and much less commonly soy, wheat and egg. The longer list of foods relates to IgE mediated food allergies, while this shorter list is for delayed allergies. If your child reacts to these foods during weaning, the delay could be from a matter of hours to 2–3 days.

It is worth, therefore, making a note of when you introduce these foods into your child's diet and any changes in appearance or behaviour in the following 2–3 days.

Reactions to other major allergens such as nuts, fish and eggs are generally immediate so you will know straight away after your child has eaten them if there is a problem.

For foods containing common allergens where delayed allergy is suspected therefore:

Detect: Wait three days to allow symptoms to show.

Define: What were the symptoms? Include visible ones, such as rashes, and invisible ones, such as unsettled behaviour.

Document: Write it all down in your food and symptoms diaries (see pages 55 and 185).

The selection of food to use will be guided by your child's food allergies.

Time of day

Introduce new foods during the morning or early afternoon because should an adverse reaction occur during these times, it will cause the least amount of disruption to your baby's sleep and routine.

Get creative

Within the remit of your child's emerging allergies, try to aim to introduce as wide a variety of foods as possible into the diet and zone in on replacement foods that are nutrient-rich. At this stage it is important to learn to recognise and read food labels (see pages 80–86). Your dietician will be able to help you with this.

Follow the weaning books, which cover stages one, two and three of weaning and adapt the advice given where possible. Trying new tastes and textures in this early weaning stage up to one year is a crucial learning experience but when your child has a food allergy, offering variety can be difficult. Your child can then end up eating the same limited selection of foods based on what has been tolerated in the past. So how do you offer variety when food choices are limited?

When food type cannot be varied, try varying other aspects of your child's food, such as the texture and flavour. Below are a few suggestions:

- Offer variety within a food group. So if your child can eat carrot, offer other root vegetables such as parsnip, yam, potato, radish and sweet potato.
- Offer the foods your child can eat in different forms. Try boiled, mashed, puréed, grilled and roasted.
- Use herbs and spices to experiment with flavours.
- Combine the foods your baby can eat.

As with all children, try to make food a social, fun experience. All the members of your family can eat non-allergenic meals together to reduce any sense of exclusion or difference for the child with allergies.

Cook with your child to increase her sense of control and interest in – and confidence with – food. If you grow your own food, it is fun for your child to join in and learn. Grow vegetables, blackberries, strawberries and herbs.

To keep your child's interest, vary the way she is offered food. Try finger foods as well as purées. Always offer praise and encouragement to create a relaxed and happy mealtime.

Don't give up!

Always remember that all is not lost if your child's weaning experience has not been varied. You can try new flavours later on, once she's a toddler. At this stage it may take longer and need many more attempts before your child accepts and gains a preference for a new food, but it is worth persevering. Weaning an allergic child is a slower process, but with patience, acceptance, imagination and dedication, it does not need to be any less adventurous or exciting.

CHAPTER 15
Related Foods and Reactions

Once your child has reacted to one food, it is important to know what else he may react to, especially during the weaning process. This section will aim to bring some clarity to this by looking at the major allergens and their food groups, cross-reactions and additives.

Peanuts
● ●

Peanuts are related to legumes or beans, such as peas and soy, although most peanut allergy sufferers can tolerate other beans. However, despite being a different family, the most common allergies associated with peanut are tree nuts (see Page 192). Around 30–40 per cent of peanut allergic children will react to tree nuts. Some families have a policy of avoiding all nuts due to the risk of cross-contamination while others, under careful guidance from their doctors, will introduce select tree nuts into their diets, just at home, where the risk of cross-contamination can be better managed. Outside the home, all nuts are avoided. A similar approach can be taken in children with specific tree nut allergies who can often tolerate either peanut or other tree nuts.

About 25 per cent of peanut allergic children will react to sesame while 4 per cent will react to lupin – a pea whose flour is sometimes used in baked goods, particularly on the continent.

Tree Nuts
. . . .

Tree nuts are not related to peanuts and an allergy to one type of tree nut does not necessarily mean an allergy to others. Tree nuts include almond, Brazil, cashew, chestnut, hazelnut, pecan, macadamia, pistachio and walnut. The most common tree nut allergy is cashew, which almost always cross-reacts with pistachio. In many shop-bought products and in tree nut oils there is a risk of cross-contamination, so it is often advised that all nuts be avoided. As discussed above, select nuts may be introduced at home but this needs to be tailored to the individual and may require the nuts that are suspected to be fine to be tested first under medical supervision.

It is worth noting that coconut, water chestnut, butternut and nutmeg are not nuts. Coconut does share some proteins with walnut but coconut allergy is rare. Pine nut is also not a nut (it's a seed) so is usually fine but be careful to look for cashew or walnut added to pesto.

Seeds
. . . .

Sesame and poppy seeds can cause a severe allergic reaction. Other seeds include sunflower, rapeseed and flaxseed. The oils of these seeds contain variable amounts of protein and are often tolerated, especially when used in cooking. Sesame is the most common seed to cause allergies and is commonly associated with peanut allergy, rather than problems with other seeds. If you want your child to have other seeds, your doctor may wish to do some allergy tests first.

Eggs and Vaccines

It is assumed that a child who is allergic to chicken eggs will also react to other bird eggs. Although this has not been extensively studied, it is best to avoid giving your child any eggs. Very few egg-allergic children have a problem with fish egg (such as cod roe) so there is no reason to avoid these unless you have experienced a problem. However, 20–30 per cent of egg-allergic children develop peanut allergy, usually during infancy. This needs to be checked for by your doctor, especially as simply avoiding peanut in case of allergy is not the answer. There is some evidence that avoidance may increase the chances of allergy. If your child has an egg allergy, ask your doctor to test for peanut allergy and if the test is negative, consider introducing peanut into the diet. Egg lecithin is sometimes used as an emulsifier and can be used to prevent sticking, for example in non-stick cooking spray. Always check the type of emulsifier used and avoid if egg based.

Egg is also used in some childhood vaccines, such as the MMR, flu and yellow fever jab. It is now known that the MMR vaccine is safe for children with egg allergy. With flu jabs, it will depend on the egg content so discuss this with your child's allergist and ask for approval in writing to have the vaccine if it is safe for your child, ideally in your child's red personal health record book, to avoid unnecessary confusion or delay when your child goes to the practice nurse for his injection. Yellow fever vaccine also contains egg so if your child needs this, he will need a referral to a specialist allergy centre for the vaccine to be administered carefully under supervision (sometimes in divided doses).

Cow's Milk

As previously discussed (see page 179), a child who is allergic to cow's milk is highly likely to react to other mammal milk such as sheep's or goat's milk. Although it rarely happens, some children can also react to beef, especially if it has not been cooked properly, as it can retain some cow's milk proteins. Children with delayed allergy to milk are also at increased risk of allergy to soy, which is thus usually avoided during infancy.

Soy

Soy is a legume and people with a soy allergy do not usually have a reaction to other beans. Soy oil has very low levels of soy protein and soy lecithin (used instead of egg lecithin), a fatty derivative of soy has trace protein so both of these products can usually be tolerated by a person with soy allergy. Discuss this with your child's dietician.

Wheat

Children with a wheat allergy are sometimes also allergic to other grains. Spelt is wheat and causes the same reaction. Rice is not closely related to wheat, so can often be tolerated.

Wheat is made up of albumin, globulin, gliadin and gluten. Gluten is a component of wheat. The majority of allergic reactions to wheat are caused by albumin and globulin. The difference is important especially when reading food labels. A gluten-free item will not always be wheat free, while a wheat-free item may contain gluten from other sources (such as barley) so may be suitable for wheat-allergic children but not those with Coeliac disease.

Coeliac disease is different to a wheat allergy, as it is an autoimmune disease triggered by the gluten in grains such as wheat, barley and rye. Coeliac disease sufferers must avoid all gluten, which can be hidden in soups, sauces and even cosmetics.

Fish

With fish allergy, if there is an allergy to one type of finned fish, the doctor will often advise you to avoid all finned fish. However, sometimes a person can be allergic to just one type of fish and tolerate others and sometimes the tinned version of the fish, such as salmon or tuna, can be tolerated, but the fresh cooked fish not tolerated. Being allergic to fish does not mean your child will be allergic to shellfish – ask for tests.

Shellfish

Crustacean shellfish, including lobster, shrimp and crab, are well known for causing severe reactions and the majority of sufferers will react to more than one type. Molluscs or bivalves, such as scallops, clam and oyster, are a different family, as are cephalopods, such as squid and octopus. Potentially your child can be allergic to one but not the other of these families, although most children with a shellfish allergy will avoid them all. If seafood is an important part of your diet, you may wish to define the allergies more precisely.

Fruits and Vegetables

The most common allergy with fruit and vegetables is Oral Allergy Syndrome (see page 8). These reactions are usually mild and can be to just one fruit or to many fruits and vegetables. Often the fruit and vegetables can be tolerated when cooked. Common examples include apple, pear, plum and carrot.

Meats

Meat allergy is relatively uncommon. A person who is allergic to chicken may be more likely to react to other forms of poultry, such as turkey, and a person allergic to mammalian meats may react to them all (beef, pork and lamb).

Additives

Allergy to food additives is uncommon because many do not contain proteins or only in very small quantities. However, certain food additives that are from natural sources, such as soybean, corn and beets, do contain proteins and these are more likely to cause an allergic reaction. Chemical additives can also cause non-allergic reactions (typically benzoates or azo dyes), but again these are not common.

Home-cooking
• •

The reason that the parents of children with food allergies home-cook most of their child's food is because of the risk from cross-contamination when eating out and from confused food labelling on bought, processed food.

Zach has multiple food allergies. When he was first diagnosed, it took me months to accept that home-cooking was the safest option for him. I couldn't cook and, more importantly, really didn't enjoy cooking. It was a huge learning curve, but one that I have taken and had a few laughs at my own expense along the way. If I can do it, believe me, so can you! After a few years of practice, I feel established as a very competent allergy-free cook and am able to provide healthy alternatives and delicious treats and snacks for my little boy.

CHAPTER 16

Recipes

This book is not a cookbook, but it does equip you with the information that you need to be able to make your own allergy-free recipes. In the Resources section (see Baking page 257) there are also some links to blogs and other books, which contain amazing allergy-free recipes that you can follow.

When I was going through the process of Zach being diagnosed with multiple food allergies, ease became all-important. I didn't have time to be searching for allergy-free recipes. I needed to have some essential basic recipes available to me for everyday meals as well as the big celebration events in the year. To help get you started on some celebration baking and to make the first few years of life easier, this chapter contains a few recipes that work well and children love. These recipes are mainly dairy-, egg-, nut- and gluten-free and where they are not, alternatives have been suggested. Please check each recipe so that you know that it is safe for your child.

The recipes cover the occasions that you may celebrate with your child from Christmas to Easter and of course birthdays. I've also included a great cupcake recipe that can be adapted for any occasion given the right decoration, as well as some essential snack and lunchbox ideas.

Ingredients
• •

- I use Doves Farm flours, baking powder and xanthan gum as these are all made without the major allergens. However, other brands are available.

- I also use Pure Sunflower, available in major supermarkets.

- In one of the pastry recipes I have used coconut oil because it has a consistency similar to butter and it is very good for you. However, it is expensive and has a strong flavour, so I have also included an alternative.

- Baking Block is used in some of the recipes as again it is nutritious, made of palm oil and rapeseed oil. This is available in supermarkets. Please check the labels, however, because some brands are labelled 'may contain milk'.

- Some of the recipes use icing sugar. Tate & Lyle's version says 'may contain egg' so please avoid if your child has an egg allergy. Marks & Spencer's own-brand icing sugar is allergen-free.

- Be careful to buy gluten-free baking powder as well because baking powder contains wheat.

- Some cocoa powder brands carry a 'may contain milk' allergy alert.

- Lyle's golden syrup is gluten-free but please check others.

Caution: Always read the labels of any ingredients each time that you buy them to double check for allergens.

Ingredient Substitutes

Below are some ingredient substitutes which can be used to enable you to learn to cook allergy-free.

Egg

In the recipes below, I have tended to favour the use of egg replacer with xanthan gum as I found that it works well. However, do try the alternatives as each adds a different quality to the recipe.

For one egg:

- 2 tbsp applesauce and ½ tsp baking powder.
- 2 tbsp water, 1 tbsp oil, 2 tsp baking powder.
- 1 tsp baking powder, 1 tbsp water, 1 tbsp vinegar.
- 1 packet gelatin, 2 tbsp warm water.
- 1 tsp yeast dissolved in ¼ cup water.
- Ground linseed (also known as flaxseed) – mix two tablespoons with a small amount of water or dairy-free milk.
- Ener-G egg replacer – mix one teaspoon with two tablespoons cold water or substitute milk and a pinch of xanthan gum.
- ½ mashed banana and ½ tsp baking powder.

Dairy

- Replace cow's milk with any plant, rice, hemp or nut milk.
- Use 9.5 g (⅓ oz) of soya, canola or sunflower margarine or 1 tbsp oil for 15 g (½ oz) of 'butter'.
- Use half-vegetable lard or Baking Block and half sunflower margarine.
- Use dairy-free cheese.
- Buttermilk – mix 1 tbsp lemon juice with 240 ml (8½ fl oz) substitute milk and allow to stand for 10 minutes for 240 ml (8½ fl oz) of buttermilk.
- Vegan yoghurt or soya cream for cream.

Gluten

Gluten-free flour, plus xanthan gum.

Nuts

Sunflower seeds are a good replacement for peanuts or tree nuts in baking.

Celebrations and Occasions

Christmas cake

Egg-free, dairy-free, nut-free and gluten-free

Serves 8–10

This is a delicious fruit cake, which can be made as a fruit loaf or styled into a Christmas cake. Please remember to check the ingredients of any edible decorations that you use on your cake for allergens.

INGREDIENTS

200 g (8 oz) gluten-free self-raising flour

2 level tsp mixed spice

1 level tsp gluten-free baking powder

100 g (4 oz) dairy-free margarine

100 g (4 oz) soft light brown sugar

½ medium banana, mashed

2 tbsp substitute milk

100g (4oz) dried raisins

100g (4oz) dried cranberries

TO DECORATE (OPTIONAL)

> 1 kg packet of ready-to-roll icing (I used Dr Oetker White Regal Ice Ready to Roll Icing)
>
> Christmas cake decorations

WHAT TO DO

Grease a loaf tin and line the bottom with baking parchment. Preheat the oven to 160°C/325°F/Gas mark 3. Sift the flour, spice and baking powder into a mixing bowl. Melt the margarine and sugar on a low heat and add to the bowl. Mash the banana with the milk and add that to the bowl. Add the fruit and mix well. Pour into the loaf tin. Bake in the oven for 1 hour or until a skewer comes out clean. Allow to cool in the tin before transferring to a wire rack.

For a Christmas cake, pour the mixture into a 23 cm (9 in) cake tin, cover with ready-to-roll white icing and decorate with Christmas decorations. I used Renshaw's Ready to Roll icing. It is not suitable for nut allergy sufferers due to the manufacturing methods. The Co-Op brand is suitable but please check the label.

> Prep Time: 10 mins
>
> Cooking Time: 1 hr
>
> Decorating Time: 10 mins
>
> Total Time: 1 hr 20 mins

Gingerbread people

Egg-free, dairy-free, nut-free and gluten-free

Makes up to 24 mini people, depending on the cutter size. Any unused dough can be kept in the freezer for up to one month.

This is an easy recipe for gingerbread men, but you can experiment with any shapes you want. Add a ribbon and they become Christmas decorations to hang on the tree or gifts for your favourite people.

INGREDIENTS

> 350 g (12 oz) gluten-free plain flour, plus extra for rolling out
>
> 1 tsp bicarbonate of soda
>
> 2 tsp ground ginger
>
> 1 tsp ground cinnamon
>
> ¼ tsp xanthan gum, plus a pinch
>
> 125 g (4½ oz) sunflower margarine
>
> 175 g (6 oz) light soft brown sugar
>
> 1 tsp Ener-G egg replacer
>
> 2 tbsp substitute milk
>
> 4 tbsp golden syrup

TO DECORATE

> Writing icing
>
> Cake decorations

WHAT TO DO

Sift the flour, bicarbonate of soda, ginger and cinnamon into a bowl. Add the ¼ tsp of xanthan gum. Pour into the bowl of a food processor. Add the margarine and blend until the mix looks like breadcrumbs. Stir in the sugar. With a small hand whisk or fork combine the egg replacer, milk substitute and a pinch of xanthan gum until it is a thick consistency without lumps. Add the egg replacer mix and golden syrup to the food processor and pulse until the mixture clumps together. Remove the dough, wrap in clingfilm and leave in the fridge for 15 minutes.

Preheat the oven to 180°C/350°F/Gas mark 4 and line two baking trays with baking parchment. Roll the dough out to a 0.5 cm (¼ in) thickness on a lightly floured surface. Using cutters, cut out the gingerbread men shapes and place on the baking trays, leaving a gap between them. Use something with a rounded pointy end (I use the end of a whisk!) to carve eyes, a smile and a hole where you would like to thread a ribbon. The dough is quite fragile, so arrange the shapes on the baking trays carefully.

Bake for 12–15 minutes, or until lightly golden-brown. Leave on the trays for 10 minutes and then move to a wire rack to finish cooling. When cooled, decorate with the writing icing and cake decorations. Pile them together and tie with a ribbon, or thread your ribbon through the hole and hang on your tree.

Prep Time: 10 mins

Cooking Time: 15 mins

Decorating Time: 10 mins

Total Time: 35 mins

Birthdays

. . . .

Sponge cake

Egg-free, dairy-free, nut-free and gluten-free

Serves 8–10

INGREDIENTS

4 tsp Ener-G Egg Replacer

8 tbsp substitute milk

1 tsp xanthan gum, plus a pinch

300 g (10 oz) gluten-free self-raising flour

2 tsp gluten-free baking powder

300 g (10 oz) caster sugar

140 g (5 oz) Cookeen

140 g (5 oz) dairy-free margarine

6 tbsp substitute milk

1 tsp vanilla essence

TO DECORATE

Raspberry jam

Fresh berries

Icing sugar

WHAT TO DO

Preheat the oven to 180°C/350°F/Gas mark 4. Line two 18 cm (7 in) cake tins with baking parchment. In a small bowl, hand whisk together the egg replacer, 8 tablespoons of milk and pinch of xanthan gum. Mix the flour, 1 teaspoon xanthan gum and baking powder. Add the egg replacer mix and the sugar and mix. Add the Cookeen (at room temperature), margarine, 6 tablespoons of milk and vanilla essence. Whisk on a medium speed until the mixture is creamy. Bake in the oven for 35–40 minutes. Remove from the oven and transfer to a wire rack to cool.

When the two sponge layers are cooled, spread one cake layer with jam and add the fresh berries. Place the other cake layer on top and gently press down. Add another thin layer of jam to the top of the cake and decorate with fresh berries. Dust with icing sugar.

Prep Time: 15 mins

Cooking Time: 40 mins

Total Time: 55 mins

Chocolate cake

Egg-free, dairy-free, nut-free and gluten-free

Serves 8–10

INGREDIENTS

> 280 g (10 oz) gluten-free plain flour
>
> ½ tsp xanthan gum
>
> 55 g (2 oz) cocoa powder
>
> 200 g (7 oz) caster sugar
>
> 1 tsp bicarbonate of soda
>
> 150 ml (5 fl oz) orange juice
>
> 150 ml (5 fl oz) cold water
>
> 240 ml (8 fl oz) sunflower oil
>
> 1 tsp vanilla essence

FOR THE ICING

> 120 g (4 oz) dairy-free margarine
>
> 8 tbsp cocoa powder
>
> Splash of substitute milk
>
> Icing sugar

WHAT TO DO

Preheat the oven to 180°C/350°F/Gas mark 4. Mix the dry ingredients in a bowl. Mix the wet ingredients in a separate bowl. Gradually add the wet to the dry ingredients, whisking as you add. Pour into an 18 cm (7 in) round cake tin.

Bake for 45–50 minutes until a skewer comes out clean. Allow to cool before icing.

FOR THE ICING

Whisk the margarine, cocoa powder and splash of milk on a medium speed until the consistency is smooth and thick. Add icing sugar to taste and whisk on a medium speed. Remove the cake from the tin, allow to cool and use a spatula to smooth the icing over the cake.

Prep Time: 15 mins

Cooking Time: 50 mins

Total Time: 1 hr 5 mins

Valentine's Day

Red velvet cupcakes with vanilla icing
Egg-free, dairy-free, nut-free and gluten-free

Makes 12 cupcakes

INGREDIENTS

1 tsp Ener-G egg replacer

120 ml (4 fl oz) dairy-free substitute milk, plus 2 tbsp

½ tsp xanthan gum, plus a pinch

60 g (2 oz) dairy-free margarine

150 g (5 oz) caster sugar

20 g (1 oz) cocoa powder

40 ml (1½ fl oz) red food colouring

½ tsp vanilla extract

150 g (5 oz) gluten-free plain flour

½ tsp bicarbonate of soda

1½ tsp white vinegar

FOR THE ICING

300 g (10 oz) icing sugar

20 g (1 oz) dairy-free margarine

1 tsp vanilla essence

Splash of substitute milk

WHAT TO DO

Preheat the oven to 170°C/335°F/Gas mark 3. In a small bowl, combine the egg replacer with 2 tablespoons of substitute milk. Mix well and add a pinch of xanthan gum. Put the margarine and sugar into a bowl and whisk on a medium speed until light, fluffy and well mixed. Turn the whisk up to a high speed and add the egg replacer mixture. Whisk until well mixed. In a separate bowl, mix together the cocoa powder, red food colouring and vanilla extract to make a very thick, dark paste. Add this to the margarine mixture and mix thoroughly until evenly combined and coloured. Turn the whisk down to a slow speed and slowly add the 120 ml (4 fl oz) of substitute milk. Sift the flour in and ½ teaspoon of xanthan gum and whisk until everything is well incorporated. Turn the whisk up to a high speed and beat until you have a smooth, even mixture. Turn the whisk down to a low speed and add the bicarbonate of soda and vinegar. Whisk until well mixed, then turn up the speed again and whisk for a couple more minutes.

To make the icing, whisk the icing sugar and margarine together in a bowl on medium-slow speed until the mixture comes together and is well mixed. Turn the whisk up to a medium-high speed. Add the vanilla essence and splash of milk substitute. Continue until the icing is light and fluffy – at least five minutes. Spoon the mixture into 12 paper cases in a cupcake tray until two-thirds full and bake in the oven for 20–25 minutes, or until the sponge bounces back when touched. A skewer inserted in the centre should come out clean. Leave the cupcakes to cool slightly in the tin before turning out on to a wire cooling rack to cool completely. When the cupcakes are cold, spoon or pipe the icing on top.

Prep Time: 20 mins
Cooking Time: 25 mins
Total Time: 45 mins

Heart-shaped shortbread biscuits
Egg-free, dairy-free, nut-free and gluten-free

Makes 8 biscuits

INGREDIENTS

  125 g (4 oz) dairy-free margarine

  55 g (2 oz) caster sugar

  180 g (6 oz) gluten-free plain flour

  1 tsp substitute milk

  Icing sugar, for sprinkling

WHAT TO DO

Preheat the oven to 190°C/375°F/Gas mark 5. Whisk the margarine and sugar together until smooth. Stir in the flour and milk to get a smooth paste. Using your hands, knead the dough into a ball. Cover in clingfilm and place in the fridge for 30 minutes. Roll out to about 1 cm (½ in) thick and use a heart cutter to create heart-shaped biscuits. Bake in the oven for 20 minutes until pale golden brown. Transfer to a wire rack to cool. Sprinkle with icing sugar.

  Prep Time: 40 mins

  Cooking Time: 20 mins

  Total Time: 1 hr

Easter

Lemon cupcakes with icing chicks
Egg-free, dairy-free and gluten-free

Makes 12 cupcakes

INGREDIENTS

    2 tsp Ener-G egg replacer

    4 tbsp substitute milk

    ½ tsp and 2 pinches of xanthan gum

    125 g (4½ oz) gluten-free self-raising flour

    1 tsp gluten-free baking powder

    125 g (4½ oz) caster sugar

    125 g (4½ oz) sunflower margarine

    Finely grated zest of 1 small lemon

    1 tbsp substitute milk

FOR THE ICING

    300 g (10 oz) icing sugar

    50 g (2 oz) sunflower margarine

    Juice of 1 small lemon

FOR THE CHICKS

    1 pack of yellow fondant icing for the body and head

    1 pack of orange for the beak and feet

    1 pack of black for the eyes

Note: I used Renshaw's Professional Ready to Roll Icing. It is not suitable for nut-allergy sufferers due to manufacturing methods. The Co-Op brand is suitable but please check the labels.

WHAT TO DO

Preheat the oven to 180°C/350°F/Gas mark 4. Combine the egg replacer, 4 tablespoons of milk and 2 pinches of xanthan gum in a small bowl. Leave to one side. Sift the flour and baking powder into a mixing bowl, add the sugar and ½ teaspoon xanthan gum. Add the margarine and whisk. Grate the zest of one lemon into the mixing bowl and add a tablespoon of substitute milk. Add the egg replacer mixture and continue to whisk on a medium-slow speed, until the mixture comes together and is well mixed. Place the paper cases in 12-hole cupcake tray and fill to three-quarters full. Place in the oven for 20–25 minutes until a skewer comes out clean from the centre or until they spring back when gently touched.

To make the icing, whisk the icing sugar and margarine together in a bowl. Turn the whisk up to medium-high speed. Slowly add the lemon juice. Continue until the icing is light and fluffy – at least five minutes. Allow the cupcakes to cool, then transfer to a rack. Spoon the icing on the top.

To make the chicks, roll two balls of yellow icing, one slightly smaller than the other. Place the smaller ball on top of the larger one. Roll out the orange icing to a thin sheet and cut out three small triangles, one for the beak and two for the feet. Place the beak and feet in place then roll out two small black icing balls for eyes and attach. It may be necessary to use a bit of water to stick the icing together.

> Prep Time: 15 mins
> Cooking Time: 25 mins
> Decorating Time: 15 mins
> Total Time: 55 mins

Chocolate bunny

Egg-free, dairy-free, nut-free and gluten-free

Makes 1 bunny

INGREDIENTS

160 g (5½ oz) 'free from' dark chocolate

EQUIPMENT

80 × 65 × 20 mm bunny chocolate mould (I bought mine from www.dennycraftmoulds.co.uk but others are available)

Gold foil (www.cakecraftshop.co.uk)

Red ribbon (www.cakecraftshop.co.uk)

WHAT TO DO

Break the chocolate into a small glass or ceramic bowl. Place 5 cm (2 in) of water in to a small saucepan and bring to the boil. Place the bowl on top of the saucepan and on a medium heat allow the steam from the water to melt the chocolate. Once melted pour into the bunny mould. Place in the fridge overnight. Gently turn the bunny out of the mould onto a clean flat surface then carefully wrap in foil, taking care to smooth down the contours. Wrap a ribbon around the neck. Store in the fridge.

Prep Time: 15 mins, plus store in the fridge overnight

Decorating Time: 10 mins

Total time: 25 mins

THE ALLERGY-FREE BABY & TODDLER BOOK

Pancake Day
• •

Pancakes with sugar and lemon
Egg-free, dairy-free, nut-free and gluten-free

Makes 4 pancakes

INGREDIENTS

> 115 g (4 oz) gluten-free plain flour
>
> 2 tsp gluten-free baking powder
>
> 1 tsp caster sugar
>
> 270 ml (9 fl oz) soya or rice milk
>
> 2 tbsp water
>
> 2 tbsp sunflower oil, plus extra for cooking
>
> Juice from 1 lemon
>
> Caster sugar to sprinkle

WHAT TO DO

Sieve the flour into a bowl or large jug. Add the baking powder and sugar. Gradually whisk in the substitute milk, water and oil to make a smooth creamy batter. Heat a little oil around a frying pan, then turn the heat down to medium and pour in roughly 3 tablespoons of batter. Once the batter has bubbled and set, flip the pancake over and fry the other side. Using a fork, juice one lemon and drizzle some over the pancake. Sprinkle with sugar to taste.

> Prep Time: 10 mins
>
> Cooking Time: 15 mins
>
> Total Time: 25 mins

Bonfire Night
●●

Treacle flapjack bites
Egg-free, dairy-free, nut-free and gluten-free

Makes 24 bites

INGREDIENTS
> 225 g (8 oz) gluten-free pure oats (I use Bob's Red Mill Pure Oats)
> 55 g (2 oz) dried fruit (I use cranberries and raisins but any will do)
> 55 g (2 oz) linseeds
> 170 g (6 oz) baking block or 85 g (3½ oz) dairy-free margarine
> and 85 g (3½ oz) Cookeen
> 75 g (3 oz) muscovado sugar
> 2 tbsp Lyle's black treacle

WHAT TO DO
Preheat the oven to 180°C/350°F/Gas mark 4. Mix the oats, fruit and linseeds in a bowl. Place the baking block or margarine and Cookeen, sugar and treacle in a small saucepan and heat on a low heat, stirring continuously until melted. Add this to the bowl and mix well together with a wooden spoon. Line an 18 cm (7 in) square baking tray with baking parchment. Tip the mixture into the baking tray and press down firmly with a spoon until compact. Cook for 15–20 minutes until golden brown. Wait until cooled and cut into 2.5 cm (1 in) bite-sized pieces.

> Prep Time: 10 mins
> Cooking Time: 20 mins
> Total Time: 30 mins

Black treacle and banana loaf
Egg-free, dairy-free, nut-free and gluten-free

Serves 10–12

INGREDIENTS

>   225 g (8 oz) gluten-free plain flour
>
>   1 tbsp gluten-free baking powder
>
>   3 tbsp Lyle's black treacle
>
>   85 g (3 oz) dark brown, unrefined soft sugar
>
>   85 g (3 oz) dairy-free margarine
>
>   1 banana, mashed
>
>   150 ml (5 fl oz) substitute milk

WHAT TO DO

Preheat the oven to 180°C/350°F/Gas mark 4. Combine the flour and baking powder in a large mixing bowl. Melt the treacle, sugar and margarine in a small saucepan on a low heat. Add the treacle mixture to the flour and combine with a wooden spoon. Add the banana and combine. Add the milk and mix well

Line an 18 cm (7 in) loaf tin with baking parchment. Pour the mixture into the tin and place on the middle shelf in the oven. Bake for 30 minutes or until a skewer comes out clean from the middle. Leave to cool before cutting into small slices.

>   Prep time: 15 mins
>
>   Cook time: 30 mins
>
>   Total time: 45 mins

Party Food
. . . .

Chocolate cupcakes with vanilla icing
Egg-free, dairy-free, nut-free and gluten-free

Makes 12 cupcakes

INGREDIENTS

>   1 tsp Ener-G egg replacer
>
>   120 ml (5 fl oz) plus 2 tbsp substitute milk
>
>   ½ tsp xanthan gum, plus a pinch
>
>   50 g (2 oz) sunflower margarine
>
>   150 g (5 oz) caster sugar
>
>   20 g (1 oz) cocoa powder
>
>   ½ tsp vanilla extract
>
>   150 g (5 oz) gluten-free self-raising flour
>
>   ½ tsp bicarbonate of soda
>
>   1½ tsp white vinegar

FOR THE ICING

>   300 g (10 oz) icing sugar
>
>   50 g (2 oz) dairy-free margarine
>
>   1 tsp vanilla essence
>
>   Splash of substitute milk

TO DECORATE

>   1 packet of dairy-free chocolate buttons

WHAT TO DO

Preheat the oven to 170°C/335°F/Gas mark 3. In a small bowl, combine the egg replacer with 2 tbsp of substitute milk. Mix well and add a pinch of xanthan gum. Put the margarine and sugar in a bowl and whisk on a medium speed until light, fluffy and well mixed. Turn the whisk up to a high speed and add the egg replacer mixture. Whisk until well mixed. In a separate bowl, mix together the cocoa powder and vanilla extract to make a very thick, dark paste. Add this to the margarine mixture and mix thoroughly. Turn the whisk down to a slow speed and slowly add the 120 ml (5 fl oz) substitute milk. Slowly add the flour and ½ teaspoon of xanthan gum and whisk until everything is well incorporated. Turn the whisk up to a high speed and beat until you have a smooth, even mixture. Turn the whisk down to a low speed and add the bicarbonate of soda and vinegar. Whisk until well mixed, then turn up the speed again and whisk for a couple more minutes. Place the paper cases in a 12-hole cupcake tray, spoon the mixture into the paper cases until two-thirds full and bake in the oven for 15–20 minutes, or until the sponge bounces back when touched. A skewer inserted in the centre should come out clean.

In the meantime, to make the icing whisk the icing sugar, 50 g (2 oz) of margarine and vanilla essence together in a bowl on medium-slow speed until the mixture comes together and is well mixed. Turn the whisk up to medium-high speed. Slowly add the substitute milk and continue whisking until the icing is light and fluffy – at least five minutes. Leave the cupcakes to cool slightly in the tin before turning out on to a wire cooling rack to cool completely. When the cupcakes are cold, spoon or pipe the vanilla icing on top and decorate with dairy-free chocolate buttons.

> Prep Time: 20 mins
> Cooking Time: 20 mins
> Total Time: 40 mins

Vanilla cupcakes

Egg-free, dairy-free, nut-free and gluten-free

Makes 18 cupcakes (eat some and freeze the rest!)

This is an all-round brilliant cupcake recipe from a blog called Sweet Rosie (www.sweetrosie.wordpress.com), which I have made gluten-free. It is the most delicious and versatile recipe. Decorate it however you choose to suit the occasion.

INGREDIENTS

    1 tbsp white wine vinegar

    2 tbsp sunflower oil

    240 ml (8 fl oz) substitute milk

    230 g (8 oz) caster sugar

    255 g (9 oz) gluten-free self-raising flour

    1 tbsp gluten-free baking powder

    ½ tsp bicarbonate of soda

    1 tsp vanilla extract

FOR THE ICING

    300 g (10 oz) icing sugar

    50 g (2 oz) dairy-free margarine

    Splash of substitute milk

WHAT TO DO

Preheat the oven to 180°C/350°F/Gas mark 4. Combine the vinegar, oil and milk. Put everything else into the mixer bowl. Add the vinegar mixture. Whisk the ingredients on a medium speed. Fill the cupcake cases three-quarters full and put into the oven for 20–25 minutes until they spring back when gently touched or a skewer inserted into the centre comes out clean. Allow the cupcakes to cool, then transfer to a rack.

To make the icing, whisk the icing sugar and the margarine together in a bowl on a medium-slow speed, until the mixture comes together and is well mixed. Turn the whisk up to medium-high speed. Slowly add the substitute milk and continue whisking until the icing is light and fluffy, at least five minutes. Decorate the cupcakes if you wish.

> Prep Time: 20 mins
> Cooking Time: 25 mins
> Total Time: 45 mins

Savoury and Sweet Lunchbox Ideas

It will be a rare occasion that you will leave the house for the day without a lunchbox for your child. These lunchbox ideas are designed to make lunchtime finger food slightly more interesting and tasty and to provide your child with healthy and varied lunches. They can be eaten cold or reheated. The recipes are all quite versatile so can be easily adapted to meet your child's individual tastes and preferences. Some are ideas rather than recipes, designed to show you that despite allergies there are some tricks that can make your life easier and can stimulate your child's imagination and sense of food being fun.

Crispy breaded chicken strips
Egg-free, dairy-free, nut-free and gluten-free

Makes 3 strips

INGREDIENTS

> Olive oil
> 1 slice of gluten-free wholemeal bread
> 1 chicken breast cut into three strips

WHAT TO DO

Place a glug of olive oil in a small bowl. Using your fingers, crumble 1 slice of bread into a separate bowl. If you want finer breadcrumbs, place the bread in a food processor and whizz. Slide each chicken strip through the olive oil to cover it.

Place each strip into the breadcrumbs, coating on both sides and pressing down on to the chicken to keep the breadcrumbs in place. Heat a griddle pan on a medium heat and cook the chicken strips on both sides until the chicken is cooked through and the coating is crispy. This should take about 20 minutes.

Alternatively, place the chicken strips on a baking tray and lightly cover with olive oil. Bake in a preheated oven at 200°C/400°F/Gas mark 6 for 20 minutes. Check that the chicken is white and well cooked throughout. The breadcrumbs should be golden brown.

> Prep Time: 10 mins
> Cooking Time: 20 mins
> Total Time: 30 mins

Fish strips and polenta chips
Egg-free, dairy-free, nut-free and gluten-free

Serves a family of 3–4

INGREDIENTS

> 2 tbsp olive oil for breading the fish and 2 tbsp for greasing and
> drizzling
> 350 g (12 oz) skinless cod fillets (or other white fish)
> 2 slices of gluten-free wholemeal bread
> Salt and pepper to season

FOR THE POLENTA CHIPS

    Olive oil

    500 g (17½ oz) polenta block

    Salt and pepper to season

WHAT TO DO

Preheat the oven to 200°C/400°F/Gas mark 6. Lightly grease a small baking tray with olive oil. Slice the cod fillets into strips approximately 2.5 × 7 cm (1 in × 3 in). Place the bread in a blender and pulse until the mixture is breadcrumb consistency. Season with salt and pepper and then place the crumbs on a plate. Pour 2 tablespoons olive oil into a small bowl. Take each cod strip and dip into the oil, then transfer to the bread bowl, turning the strips over and gently pushing the bread on to the fish until it is mostly covered. Place on the baking tray.

For the polenta chips, lightly grease a small baking tray with olive oil. Slice the polenta block into chip shapes approximately 1 cm (½ in) thick. Drizzle the chips with olive oil and season with salt and pepper. Bake in the oven, along with the fish for 20–25 minutes. Halfway through baking, move the fish and chips around the trays with a spatula to ensure even cooking.

    Prep Time: 20 mins

    Cooking Time: 25 mins

    Total Time: 45 mins

Mini pasties

Egg-free, dairy-free, nut-free and gluten-free

Makes 10–12 pasties

INGREDIENTS

    100 g (3½ oz) Maris Piper potatoes, peeled and cut into chunks

    100 g (3½ oz) carrots, peeled and chopped

100 g (3½ oz) tinned sweetcorn

2 tbsp olive oil

¼ tsp cumin seeds

1 onion, peeled and chopped

¼ tsp ground coriander

FOR THE PASTRY

300 g (10½ oz) wholemeal gluten-free plain flour

2 tsp olive oil

6–7 tbsp water

WHAT TO DO

Preheat the oven to 180°C/350°F/Gas mark 4. For the filling, boil the potatoes in a pan of boiling water for about 10–15 minutes, or until soft. Drain and roughly mash them. Meanwhile, bring another pan of water to the boil and cook the carrots for 5 minutes or until cooked. Add the sweetcorn and cook for a further couple of minutes. Drain and set aside. Heat the olive oil in a pan, add the cumin seeds and fry them until you start to smell them, then add the onion and continue to fry for 6–7 minutes until the onion is soft. Add the coriander, and the carrots and sweetcorn and continue to cook for a minute or two. Add this mixture to the mashed potatoes and mush together with your hands. This is easier to do if your hands are wet.

Put the flour, oil and 6–7 tablespoons of water into a bowl and mix well with your hands into a ball. Do not knead. Lightly flour a surface and roll out the dough until it is about 3 mm (⅛ in) thick. Using a circle pastry cutter, cut the pastry into circles of about 7 cm (½ in) diameter. Put approximately 1 tablespoon of the mixture into the centre of the circle, fold in half to make a package and pinch the edges together to seal. Repeat the process until all of the pastry has been used up. Place on a baking tray and put in the oven. Bake for 15–20 minutes, turning them once halfway through cooking until lightly browned.

Prep Time: 30 mins

Cooking Time: 20 mins

Total Time: 50 mins

Mini tuna kebabs

Egg-free, dairy-free, nut-free and gluten-free

Makes about 20

INGREDIENTS

7 or 8 Maris Piper potatoes, peeled and chopped into small pieces

1 × 160 g (5½ oz) tin tuna in sunflower oil

1 medium onion, peeled and finely chopped

3 tbsp sunflower oil

1 tsp garlic powder

1 tsp ground ginger

Pinch of turmeric

½ tsp ground coriander

1 tsp ground cumin

2 tbsp water

WHAT TO DO

Cook the potatoes in boiling water for 6–7 minutes or until soft. Drain and flake the tuna into a small bowl. Place the onion in a medium saucepan. Add 2 tablespoons of oil, and the garlic, ginger, turmeric, coriander and cumin and cook on a low heat until the onion is softened. Add 2 tablespoons water to the pan and stir. Turn the heat off. Once cooled, mash the potatoes. Allow all ingredients to cool, then combine the tuna, onion mixture and mashed potato into a doughy mixture in a bowl. Form into palm-sized flat discs in your hands and then gently roll out into a sausage shape. The key is to keep the kebabs small. Fry in 1 tablespoon sunflower oil, on a moderate heat, turning gently so all sides are cooked and golden brown – approximately 10 minutes. Remove from the pan, place on kitchen roll and allow to cool.

> Prep Time: 30 mins
> Cooking Time: 10 mins
> Total Time: 40 mins

Thai sticky rice

Egg-free, dairy-free, nut-free and gluten-free.
Eat rice within 24 hours of cooking and always store in the fridge.

Makes enough to fill 6 cupcake cases

INGREDIENTS
> 100 g (3½ oz) Thai sticky rice
> 180 ml (6 fl oz) water
> 120 ml (4 fl oz) coconut milk

WHAT TO DO
Place the rice and water into a saucepan, Bring to the boil, then cover and simmer for 10–15 minutes until the water is absorbed. Add the coconut milk to the rice. Stir and set aside in the fridge for 30 minutes. Form into balls and place in colourful cupcake cases. If you are really creative, you could make all sorts of animal faces by adding decoration to the rice. Check out www.cozi.com/live-simply/lunch-box-envy for more inspiration.

> Prep Time: 30 mins
> Cooking Time: 15 mins
> Total Time: 45 mins

Mini salmon cakes
Egg-free, dairy-free, nut-free and gluten-free

Makes 4 cakes

INGREDIENTS
- 1 × 213 g (7½ oz) tin of salmon
- 2 spring onions, finely chopped
- 1 tsp ground cumin
- Handful of finely chopped fresh coriander
- Salt and pepper to season
- 1 slice of gluten-free wholemeal bread
- 1 tbsp olive oil

WHAT TO DO

Place the salmon in a mixing bowl and use your fingertips to find and remove any small bones. Add the onions, cumin and coriander and mix well.

Season to taste with salt and pepper. Whizz the bread into breadcrumbs by pulsing through a blender. Add the breadcrumbs to the mixture and combine.

Place a heaped teaspoon of mixture into your hands, shape into a ball about the size of a golf ball and then gently flatten into a round. Heat the oil in a frying pan and place the salmon cakes in the pan for 2–3 minutes each side until golden brown. Place on kitchen roll to cool.

Prep Time: 20 minutes
Cooking Time: 3 minutes
Total Time: 23 minutes

Home-made burgers

Egg-free, dairy-free, nut-free and gluten-free

Makes 18 small burgers

INGREDIENTS

    2 tbsp rapeseed or olive oil

    1 medium onion, peeled and finely chopped

    1 garlic clove, peeled and finely chopped

    500 g (17½ oz) minced lean beef or lamb

    1–2 tsp chopped fresh thyme leaves

    1–2 tsp chopped fresh mint leaves

    Salt and pepper to season (optional)

WHAT TO DO

Heat 1 tablespoon rapeseed or olive oil in a frying pan over a medium heat. Add the onion and garlic and gently cook until softened. Put the meat in a large bowl and add the thyme and mint leaves. Add the cooked garlic and onion. Add salt and pepper if you want to season. Mix well with your hands. Cover and place in the fridge for an hour.

Form the mixture into balls about the size of a small egg for a child's burger. Squash them into a burger shape no more than 2 cm (¾ in) thick. Heat 1 tablespoon oil over a medium heat in a frying pan. Add the burgers and cook, turning until they are well browned with no pink in the middle.

    Prep Time: 15 mins (plus 60 mins chilling time)

    Cooking Time: 10 mins

    Total Time: 25 mins (1 hr 25 mins, including chilling time)

Falafel bites
Egg-free, dairy-free, nut-free and gluten-free

Makes 18

INGREDIENTS

>   1 large onion, peeled
>   2 garlic cloves, peeled
>   Small handful of fresh parsley
>   1 × 410 g (14 oz) tin chickpeas, drained and rinsed
>   1½ tsp ground cumin
>   1½ tsp ground coriander
>   2 tbsp gluten-free plain flour
>   3½ tbsp olive oil
>   Salt and pepper to season

WHAT TO DO

Place 2 tablespoons of olive oil into a frying pan and heat on a medium heat. Finely chop the onion, garlic and parsley and place in a blender. Add the chickpeas, cumin, coriander, flour and remaining oil. Whizz together until well combined. Season to taste. Use a teaspoon to place a golf-ball sized amount in your hand. Roll it gently into a ball and place in the pan. Fry for 5–7 minutes until golden brown. Place on kitchen roll to cool.

>   Prep Time: 10 mins
>   Cooking Time: 7 mins
>   Total Time: 17 mins

Mini pizzas
Egg-free, dairy-free, nut-free and gluten-free

Makes 4 mini pizzas

In this recipe I use shop-bought passata as it's quick, easy and allergen-free. However please check the ingredients of the brand you buy.

INGREDIENTS

FOR THE PIZZA BASE

>300 g (10½ oz) gluten-free plain flour
>1 tsp xanthan gum
>1 tsp salt
>2 tbsp olive oil, plus extra for drizzling
>1 × 7 g sachet quick yeast (I used Doves Farm)
>150 ml (5 fl oz) warm water

FOR THE TOPPING

>6–8 tbsp passata
>Toppings of your choice

WHAT TO DO

In a mixing bowl, combine the flour, xanthan gum, salt and 2 tablespoons of oil. Add the yeast. Mix with your hands while adding the water slowly until the dough is springy and non-sticky. You may not need all of the water, so do add it slowly a bit at a time. Flour a surface and then knead the dough for 5 minutes. Place the dough in a lightly oiled bowl. Cover the dough with olive oil, then cover the bowl with a clean tea towel and leave to rise somewhere warm for 30 minutes.

Preheat the oven to 200°C/400°F/Gas mark 6. Divide the dough into half and then half again. Roll the dough out thinly into rough circle shapes about 10 cm (4 in) in diameter on a lightly floured surface using a rolling pin. Lightly dust two baking trays and put the pizza bases on them.

For the topping, spoon 1–2 tablespoons of passata on to each base and add toppings of your choice, such as sweetcorn, cooked chicken, mushrooms, olives and substitute cheese. Drizzle with olive oil. Bake for 15–20 minutes until the base is cooked through.

Prep Time: 1 hr

Cooking Time: 20 mins

Total Time: 1 hr 20 mins

Healthy savoury flans

Egg-free, dairy-free, nut-free and gluten-free

Makes 4 flans

This is a great flan base for whichever fillings you and your child prefer. Try salmon and cheese substitute, broccoli and tomato, or the fillings below.

INGREDIENTS

FOR THE PASTRY

225 g (8 oz) gluten-free plain white flour

115 g (4 oz) coconut oil, Cookeen or baking block

4 tbsp cold water

FOR THE FILLING

Passata

4 thin slices of beef tomato

4 black olives, sliced into circles

A handful of sweetcorn for each flan

4–6 fresh basil leaves, roughly torn

4 handfuls of grated dairy-free cheese, 1 handful for each flan

Black pepper to season

Drizzle of olive oil for each flan

WHAT TO DO

Preheat the oven to 170°C/335°F/Gas mark 4. Place the flour in a mixing bowl and add the oil, Cookeen or Baking Block. Combine with a fork until the mixture is the consistency of large breadcrumbs. Add the water and combine with your hands into a dough. Cover with clingfilm and leave for 30 minutes. Grease 4 flan tins with substitute margarine.

Lightly cover a surface with flour. Divide the dough into 4 and roll each piece out until about 0.5 cm (¼ in) thick. Place each over a 7.5 cm (3 in) flan tin and trim the excess. Fork the base a few times. Spoon 2 tablespoons of passata onto the base, and add a slice of tomato, olives, sweetcorn, basil and then grated cheese. Season with black pepper and drizzle with olive oil. Repeat for the other tins. Place in the oven and cook for 20 minutes. Remove from the flan tins and allow to cool.

Prep Time: 45 mins

Cooking Time: 20 mins

Total Time: 1 hr 5 mins

Mixed berry tarts
Egg-free, dairy-free, nut-free and gluten-free

Makes 4 mini tarts

INGREDIENTS

225 g (8 oz) gluten-free plain flour

Either 100 g (4 oz) coconut oil or 50 g (2 oz) dairy-free margarine
plus 50 g (2 oz) Cookeen or alternative vegetable lard

1 tsp caster sugar

4 tbsp cold water

8 tsp raspberry or blackcurrant jam

A punnet each of fresh raspberries, blueberries and blackberries

Icing sugar

WHAT TO DO

Add the flour and coconut oil or margarine and Cookeen to a mixing bowl. Combine roughly using a fork and then rub together using your fingers until the mixture looks like breadcrumbs. Stir in the sugar. Add the water a little at a time, combining it with your hands until you have a ball. Wrap in clingfilm and chill in the fridge for 30 minutes.

Preheat the oven to 200°C/400°F/Gas mark 6. Grease 4 × 7.5 cm (3 in) flan tins with substitute margarine. Sprinkle the work surface and rolling pin with a little flour then roll the pastry out to about 3 mm (⅛ in) thick. Cut out 4 circles and line the tart tins. Prick the base of each tart once with a fork and bake for 5 minutes. Remove from the oven, spoon a teaspoon of fruit jam on to the base then stick the berries on top. Top with another teaspoon of jam and return the tarts to the oven for 10 minutes, then cool on a rack before anyone is allowed to taste – the jam will be very hot! Dust with icing sugar to serve.

Prep Time: 10 mins

Cooking Time: 15 mins

Total Time: 25 mins

Banana and honey loaf

Egg-free, dairy-free, nut-free and gluten-free

Serves 10

INGREDIENTS

125 g (4½ oz) dairy-free margarine

150 g (5 oz) caster sugar

1 tsp vanilla essence

3 very ripe bananas

190 g (6½ oz) gluten-free self-raising flour

1 tsp gluten-free baking powder

30 ml (1 fl oz) substitute milk

2 tbsp runny honey

WHAT TO DO

Preheat the oven to 170°C/340°F/Gas mark 3. Grease and line a 18 cm (7 in) loaf tin with baking parchment. Melt the margarine, sugar and vanilla essence in a saucepan on a low heat. Place the bananas in a bowl and mash with a fork. Put the flour, baking powder, milk, honey, mashed bananas and melted ingredients into a bowl and mix well. Pour into the tin. Bake for 40 minutes or until a skewer comes out clean from the centre of the loaf.

Tip: For a less bananary flavour, replace 1 banana with 2 tablespoons unsweetened applesauce.

Prep Time: 10 mins

Cooking Time: 40 mins

Total Time: 50 mins

Fresh strawberry muffins

Makes 12 muffins

All the muffin recipes are **egg-free, dairy-free, nut-free and gluten-free**.
The muffins tend to stick to cases so I grease the muffin trays themselves
and place the mixture straight in.

INGREDIENTS

    45 g (1½ oz) dairy-free margarine

    50 g (2 oz) golden granulated sugar

    225 g (8 oz) gluten-free wholemeal self-raising flour

    1 tsp vanilla extract

    100 ml (3½ fl oz) strawberry-flavoured substitute milk

    140 g (5 oz) fresh ripe strawberries, washed and stalks
       removed

WHAT TO DO

Preheat the oven to 200°C/400°F/Gas mark 6. Grease a muffin tray.
Gently heat the margarine and sugar in a small saucepan until the
margarine has melted. Do not let it simmer. Combine the flour with
the margarine and sugar mixture in a large mixing bowl. Add the
vanilla extract and mix well with a wooden spoon. Add the milk
slowly and combine. Mash the strawberries with a fork or whizz
in a blender, then fold into the mixture. Spoon the mixture to half
fill each muffin mould. Bake in the oven for 20 minutes until a
skewer comes out clean from the centre. Transfer to a wire rack and
leave to cool.

    Prep Time: 15 mins

    Cooking Time: 20 mins

    Total Time: 35 mins

Carrot and apple muffins (see page 234)

Makes 6–8 muffins

INGREDIENTS

> 45 g (1½ oz) diary-free margarine
>
> 225 g (8 oz) gluten-free plain flour
>
> 1 tbsp gluten-free baking powder
>
> 45 g (1½ oz) light brown sugar
>
> 2 tbsp sunflower seeds
>
> 180 ml (6 fl oz) dairy-free milk
>
> 1 medium carrot
>
> 1 large apple

WHAT TO DO

Preheat the oven to 200°C/400°F/Gas mark 6. Grease a muffin tray. Melt the margarine over a low heat in a saucepan. Combine the flour, baking powder and sugar in a bowl and mix well. Add the melted margarine and sunflower seeds and mix well, then add the milk and mix again. Peel and grate the carrot and the apple into the mixture in the bowl and mix well. Spoon the mixture into the muffin tray to just below the top of each mould. Bake for 30 minutes or until golden brown. Transfer to a wire rack and leave to cool.

> Prep Time: 10 mins
>
> Cooking Time: 30 mins
>
> Total Time: 40 mins

Cranberry, apple and cinnamon muffins (see page 234)

Makes 12 muffins

INGREDIENTS

    225 g (8 oz) gluten-free plain flour

    1 tbsp gluten-free baking powder

    1½ tsp ground cinnamon

    45 g (1½ oz) soft brown sugar

    45 g (1½ oz) dairy-free margarine

    2 apples, peeled and grated

    60 g (2 oz) dried, unsweetened cranberries

    180 ml (6 fl oz) substitute milk

WHAT TO DO

Preheat the oven to 200°C/400°F/Gas mark 6. Grease a muffin tray. Sift the flour, baking powder and cinnamon into a mixing bowl. Add the remaining ingredients and mix well into a thick, wet dough. Spoon into the muffin tray to just below the top of each mould. Bake for about 20 minutes until light golden brown and firm to touch.

    Prep Time: 10 mins

    Cooking Time: 20 mins

    Total Time: 30 mins

Banana and flaxseed muffins (see page 234)

Makes 12 muffins

INGREDIENTS

    225 g (8 oz) gluten-free plain flour

    1 tbsp gluten-free baking powder

    1 tsp ground cinnamon

    45 g (1½ oz) dairy-free margarine

45 g (1½ oz) flaxseeds

2 tbsp golden syrup

200 ml (7 fl oz) substitute milk

2 medium-sized ripe bananas

WHAT TO DO

Preheat the oven to 200°C/400°F/Gas mark 6. Grease a muffin tray. Combine the flour, baking powder and cinnamon in a bowl. Melt the margarine gently in a saucepan on a low heat. Grind the flaxseed using a coffee grinder or by hand with pestle and mortar. Add to the bowl. Mix the melted margarine, the golden syrup and milk in. Mash the bananas in a small bowl using a fork and add to the mixture.

Spoon the mixture into the muffin tray to just below the top of each mould. Bake for 30 minutes or until golden brown. Transfer to a wire rack to cool.

Prep Time: 10 mins

Cooking Time: 30 mins

Total Time: 40 mins

Sweet and Savoury Snacks

Cheese straws

Egg-free, dairy-free, gluten-free and nut-free

Makes 12–15 straws

INGREDIENTS

50 g (2 oz) gluten-free self-raising flour

25 g (1 oz) dairy-free margarine at room temperature

80 g (3 oz) mature dairy-free cheese (I used Red Cheddar Style Cheezly but you could also use Vegusto)

WHAT TO DO

Preheat oven to 200°C/400°F/Gas mark 6. Add all the ingredients to a mixing bowl. Use your hands to mix and knead the mixture together into one lump of dough. On a lightly floured surface, roll the dough out to about 1 cm (½ in) depth. Slice it into short straws, sized to fit your child's lunchbox. Pinch them gently along the top and sides to form into a straw shape. Bake in the oven for 10 minutes until golden brown. The dough will freeze and keep for up to a month.

> Prep Time: 10 mins
> Cooking Time: 10 mins
> Total Time: 20 mins

Home-made houmous with vegetable sticks
Egg-free, dairy-free, nut-free and gluten-free

INGREDIENTS

> 1 × 410 g (5 oz) tin chickpeas, drained and rinsed. Reserve the liquid in a separate bowl
> 1 tsp lemon juice
> Glug of olive oil
> 1 garlic clove
> ½ tsp ground cumin
> Chopped vegetables, such as carrots, cucumber and peppers to serve

WHAT TO DO

Whizz all the ingredients together in a food processor, adding more oil or water from the chickpea tin for the right consistency. Serve with a variety of chopped up vegetables.

Oat and honey cookies
Egg-free, dairy-free, nut-free and gluten-free

Makes 12 cookies

INGREDIENTS

    85 g (3 oz) baking block

    85 g (3 oz) dark brown, soft, unrefined cane sugar

    1 tbsp runny honey

    85 g (3 oz) gluten-free white self-raising flour

    85 g (3 oz) pure rolled gluten-free oats (I used Bob's Red Mill)

    1 tbsp substitute milk

WHAT TO DO

Preheat the oven to 180°C/350°F/Gas mark 4. Place baking parchment on a baking tray. Heat the baking block, sugar and honey in a small saucepan on a low heat until melted and combined. Combine the flour and oats in a large mixing bowl. Add the saucepan contents to the flour and oats and combine. Add the milk and mix well. Using a teaspoon, spoon out some mixture into your hands, form into a ball and then flatten into a round shape, ideally the size of a 50p.

    Place each round on to the tray, evenly spacing them. Place on the middle shelf of the oven and bake for 10 minutes. Allow to cool.

    Prep Time: 10 mins

    Cooking Time: 10 mins

    Total Time: 20 mins

Lemon and white chocolate biscuits with lemon zest

Egg-free, dairy-free, nut-free and gluten-free

Makes 10 biscuits

INGREDIENTS

> 140 g (5 oz) gluten-free, white plain flour
>
> 50 g (2 oz) caster sugar
>
> 50 g (2 oz) dairy-free white chocolate
>
> 85 g (3 oz) dairy-free margarine at room temperature
>
> Juice of ½ lemon
>
> Zest of 1 lemon

WHAT TO DO

Preheat the oven to 180°C/350°F/Gas mark 4. Place baking parchment on a baking tray. Combine the flour and sugar in a large mixing bowl. Place the chocolate and margarine in a bowl and melt above a saucepan of boiling water. Once melted add this to the bowl and mix until combined. Fold the lemon juice and zest into the mixture. Using a dessert spoon, place a heaped amount of biscuit mixture onto the baking parchment. Repeat until the mixture is used, spacing the mixture evenly apart. Place the baking tray in the oven and bake on the middle shelf for 15 minutes or until they become slightly golden. Remove from the oven, place on a wire rack and allow to cool.

> Prep Time: 10 mins
>
> Cooking Time: 15 mins
>
> Total Time: 25 mins

Gooey flapjacks
Egg-free, dairy-free, nut-free and gluten-free

Makes 9 flapjacks

INGREDIENTS

- 170 g (6 oz) baking block or 85 g (3 oz) dairy-free margarine and 85 g (3 oz) Cookeen
- 170 g (6 oz) light brown sugar
- 2 tbsp golden syrup (Lyle's is gluten-free)
- 225 g (8 oz) gluten-free pure oats (I used Bob's Red Mill Pure Oats)
- 25 g (1 oz) dried cranberries
- 25 g (1 oz) raisins
- 25 g (1 oz) linseeds
- 25 g (1 oz) sunflower seeds

WHAT TO DO

Heat the oven to 180°C/350°F/Gas mark 4. Melt the margarine, sugar and syrup in a saucepan on a low heat. Mix the rest of the ingredients together in a bowl. Add the melted ingredients and mix well. Line the bottom of a 20 × 20 cm (8 × 8 in) baking tray with baking parchment and then grease with sunflower margarine. Place the flapjack mix in the baking tray and press down with a spatula to bring the mixture together. Score into 9 pieces with a knife. Bake in the oven for 25–30 minutes.

Prep Time: 15 mins
Cooking Time: 30 mins
Total Time: 45 mins

Fruit ice lollies

Now your child will never miss out when she hears the ice-cream van approaching. Fill ice-lolly moulds with fruit juices, ripe fruit that has been whizzed up and fresh fruit pieces for an additive-free, healthy, hydrating lolly for those hot summer days.

To separate flavours or make lollies more exciting, buy different mould shapes and experiment with freezing different sections. Try a traffic light lolly by freezing apple juice first, then orange and lastly raspberry.

Juices can also be made in a blender and poured into a mould to be frozen. Keep a supply of fresh fruit lollies in your freezer.

Quick Ideas

Pasta portion

Freeze leftover gluten-free pasta or pasta bolognaise in tin foil for an individual portion. Remove from the freezer in the morning. Use only once and do not reheat more than once. Do not refreeze.

Shaped sandwiches

Use cookie cutters or buy sandwich cutters to make interesting shapes.

Corn on the cob slice

Boil a corn on the cob. Once cooled, slice an inch off the end to make a lunch box slice.

Steamed broccoli florets

Cut off the small florets from a head of broccoli. Rinse them and then steam until soft. Alternatively, rinse and then microwave for 30 seconds.

Chopped apple with lemon juice

A great tip that I learnt from a friend is to add lemon juice to chopped apple to prevent it browning in the lunchbox. It really does work!

Pots of raisins and sunflower and pumpkin seeds

Full of nibbly nutrients.

Cucumber stars and baby corn

Use mini biscuit cutters for the cucumber shapes. And chop the cooked baby corn for crunchy finger food.

Plain popcorn

Popcorn is a fun lunchtime treat or snack for your child. Allergen-free and tasty, make it plain or add sugar or syrup. Add a handful of popping corn to a tablespoon of olive or rapeseed oil in a small saucepan. Place the lid on and heat until all the corn has popped.

Apple boats with satsuma and raisin

A fun way to feed your child with healthy fruit as well as feeding her imagination. Cut an apple into quarters for the base of the boat and skewer the centre of each with a cocktail stick to make the mast. Thread a satsuma segment lengthways on to the cocktail stick to make the sail and top with a raisin to cover the cocktail stick point.

Fruit kebabs

Slices of your child's favourite fruits make a colourful, delightful dessert. Mango, pineapple, strawberry and banana slices work well, threaded on to a skewer and drizzled in honey.

CHAPTER 17
Final Words

As the mum of a now three-and-a-half-year-old with multiple food allergies, my main recommendations to other parents would be to try not to over-worry and to know that time changes many things for the better. When Zach was about 18 months old, I remember feeling so anxious about how to teach him about food and his allergies without being negative and filling him with fear about dangers and the food that he couldn't have. I used to think about it constantly and always felt preoccupied. However, as he has grown up, I know him better and I have found the right balance for him. He knows and accepts just enough to always ask before he eats something that is offered to him. I've done that through cooking, reading and playing. I've avoided sitting him down and talking to him. He is not anxious or fearful about it as far as I can tell and he has a great social life and lots of friends.

I would also like parents to know that they are not alone in the early months. It can be a struggle to get a diagnosis and clear help and support, but there are experts available and there are other parents struggling too. Keep going, persevere, follow your instincts and keep visiting the healthcare professionals until you are heard and until your child is properly managed. Life with allergies is an adventure, sometimes out of control, sometimes in control, but always about exploring and discovering and no less fun than the life of any adventurous young child. Below is the advice of the parents that I talked to and what they would like to pass on to you.

Trust Yourself

••

The parents who have kindly helped in the compilation of this book all said to trust your instincts. Below is more of what they said.

> *Try to share the responsibility with your partner as it can feel very overwhelming.*
>
> HANNAH, MUM OF S

> *Try to trust your instincts but also be vigilant and don't let people make you feel overprotective and neurotic. It is understandable to feel this way. Try to educate others as best you can so that people can be trusted to care for your child and don't be afraid to say no to someone or a situation where you feel your child might not be safe.*
>
> BEV, MUM OF LEVI

> *I would suggest you talk to other mums to share their concerns. I find other mums in our group can always help you feel better about things even if they can't give advice. I would recommend mums to trust their own instinct. If they think their child is allergic, avoid that food! I would also like to tell others not to torture themselves for feeding their son/daughter something that has caused a reaction (I would also like to take my own advice here).*
>
> EMMA, MUM OF HUNTER

It Will Improve

....

It is possible to live a near-enough normal life. Yes it takes a bit more effort but you become a master at reading labels and coming up with inventive meal ideas. My biggest nightmare was the thought of a milk allergy and I am managing one now quite successfully!

KATHRYN, MUM OF SAM AND HARRY

I wish I could say the scars of the experience healed as quickly as Alex's tummy did. Our bond was well and truly fractured. I resented him for taking my attention away from my daughter, for the stress that sleep deprivation caused between me and my husband, and for the fact that I had been miserable for a year. With perspective, I can see I had postnatal depression, but at the time I blamed him to some extent.

I'm conscious that this sounds very negative but it is honest and it is an honesty I can afford because now my son is the happiest, most delightful and loving child you could possibly hope to meet. It fills me with joy that we have recovered from such a fractious start and that he doesn't seem to remember my tears of anger and frustration with a baby who just wouldn't stop crying and then wouldn't stay asleep. Equally positive is that my relationship with my husband is pretty much back to how it was. We no longer snarl and gripe at each other in exhaustion and sadness, but now appreciate the family we have.

SAM, MUM OF ALEX

Get Professional Support

It appears from experience that very little is known about allergies, especially among the first line of help – the midwives, health visitors and GPs. It is my belief that a lot of Zach's suffering could have been avoided if there was more education around allergies, if his symptoms had been spotted and I had been listened to earlier. From a nutritional point of view, I realise that Zach did not receive the right amounts of nutrients when he was being weaned. This could have been prevented by better initial identification of suspected allergies in the community, shorter waiting times to see hospital-based specialists and then ongoing support and better access to these specialists, even if just for the few crucial months of weaning. With hindsight, I would have asked for more help as well. I would advise that if help is available for you just to get a break, or to go and see the healthcare professionals without your child, then that is very important and you should take it. On my own, faced with a team of professionals and managing a child, it was very difficult to ask the right questions, listen and to get a clear plan of action together. Share your concerns with those closest to you and ask them to help you. That way, there are other people that you can trust to care for your child and others who can also share the emotional burden with you.

When other parents were asked what they would like to change about their allergy experiences, responses were generally based around more information, advice and support.

Don't lose heart and insist on seeing a specialist. Before you see a health professional write everything down, be prepared – ask questions! If you are going to try eliminating something from your diet or the child's diet do it properly. So many people said to me – 'But I cut out my latte and it didn't make a difference'. It needs to be completely or there is no point. Ask for help, and ask family or friends if you need support but be clear on what they can and can't give your child. And above all – trust yourself!

EMILY, MUM OF FELIX

With healthcare professionals, be polite but bold; ask for what you want and on the whole they are happy to help. In terms of cooking – once you get your head around it, it is possible. Some nights I cook three different meals (I think the allergies have led to fussiness in Sam) but other glorious nights we all eat the same! Yes, it takes a bit more effort but the peace of mind that you know what your children are eating is priceless. Try eating out if you can if it is at all possible. Some of the bigger chains are really clued up. When it comes to other people, make it overtly obvious. Go over it again and again, don't let people off the hook otherwise they don't learn. If you are given something or served something containing the allergens, don't feel embarrassed, tell them. Try to trust and let go. It's hard, I need more help myself!

KATHRYN, MUM OF SAM AND HARRY

You have to have a bullish, positive attitude. A food allergy diagnosis is not a death sentence and there are far worse conditions that your child could have.

MEL, MUM OF E

You're not alone. If you have questions, ask. Never feel you are being overprotective of your child. You are your child's own advocate. If you want to cry or scream, do it. We all need to release the stress that comes along with dealing with food allergies.

Find a support group. It's always nice to find people that are going through similar situations. Stay strong and fight for your child. Don't let allergies run your life, but never let your guard down. Let your child know you love him daily and that you will do everything you can to help protect him.

ERICA, MUM OF EVAN

On reflection, I cannot fault the medical care we received – Alex may have been diagnosed earlier if I hadn't been so determined that it couldn't be a food issue as he was solely breastfed and had no diarrhoea/nappy rash. I am definitely not the person to look to for advice on maternal dairy-free diet and don't have much help to offer with weaning as I just avoided cow's milk protein in his diet for six months by not eating out and feeding him puréed fruit and veg. But I hope I can help by convincing people that, as dark as it feels now, it won't always be this bad and this difficult. Accurate diagnosis with a supportive medical team and accessing help from others will help this to become manageable and soon the crying will stop.

SAM, MUM OF ALEX

Trust your gut, get a second opinion and do what you think is best. Support from family and friends is really important and makes it easier to cope on the bad days. This has been incredibly hard to write down. I thought I was ready to share our story and I have used lots of tissues to write as much as I have. I hope it helps someone else.

ANNE, MUM OF HANNAH AND EDWARD

To improve living with food allergies, there should be better provisions in school/nurseries for severely allergic children. I think it should be classed as a disability and that they be give a person to be there for them if needed.

BEV, MUM OF LEVI

Other Support

I started to discover more about Zach's allergies by looking on the internet and typing in his symptoms. That led to cow's milk elimination from my diet and my first of many visits to the GP. For the families that shared their stories, most found support and information, outside of the immediate family, hugely lacking. Like me, they turned to social media and other internet sources for support.

Support from friends was great – I had lots of emotional support but found it very difficult to accept practical support in terms of looking after the boys. I had a family outreach worker who was wonderful and the most fabulous Homestart lady ever who is still a very good friend.

EMMA, MUM OF CAMERON AND DILLON

I found mum 'support' websites and blogs really useful. I also found a lot of useful American-based research as they appear to be a lot more aware of food allergies.

HANNAH, MUM OF S

So far people have been great. You will always get the odd person who will make unkind, unthinking comments but I think that it is often down to ignorance and selfishness and that these types of people would be like that in other situations too, sadly. My family and my friends have been fantastic and my mum always makes her home 'Levi safe' in preparation for our visits, so I can't ask for more than that.

BEV, MUM OF LEVI

I run my own support group here in Indiana (Michiana Food Allergy & Anaphylaxis Support) but there was not any support here locally. I turned to social media for help.

ERICA, MUM OF EVAN

While social networking sites and online helplines can be a good place to receive support from other parents, it is vital to exercise caution in terms of using them for diagnosis or interpretation of your child's symptoms. There are excellent UK-based charities, as we have previously mentioned, which offer telephone helplines and great websites where you can receive expert support and advice. Ultimately, support should be offered through your child's GP, specialist and dietician.

This book has attempted to provide some support and practical advice to help in the early years with your allergic child. While it does not claim to be a medical book or provide all of the answers, it is hoped that it will become a valuable resource for you. All the time, advances are being made in the medical field in terms of understanding and therefore being able to treat allergies comprehensively. There are those in the medical profession who are striving to educate others in order to improve your experience of diagnosis and treatment within the NHS. There is still, however, much more work to be done.

There are also more and more resources becoming available on the internet, from blogs about living with allergies to 'free from' recipes. There are recipe books as well as educational books for your child. While all of this is developing, the immediate difficulty still remains for you, as a parent, in trying to understand, determine and seek the right treatment and management approach for your child. Take the guidance in this book that suits you and that is helpful to your situation. Tailor your approach to your child and lifestyle.

As it stands at the moment, Zach is approaching school age and does not look likely to outgrow his allergies. He is also developing others. While it is a sobering reality for him and for us as his parents, it is a part of his life. Zach is not ill, he is very well, very happy and full of energy. For now, he accepts that there are things that he cannot eat while his friends can. I am aware of how I talk about allergies and how much anxiety I allow them to create for me at social events, at preschool and with family and friends, yet still sometimes I find myself welling up as I walk past the cereal or yoghurt aisle in the supermarket. However, that is my upset and not his.

Allergies do influence everything that we do as a family and all the while I am not with him I have nagging worries in the back of my mind. My role will change as he gets older and I naturally plan to love and support him through whatever the future holds. Either way, Zach is managing very well and will continue to do so in the future. Allergies are a part of his life, but not everything and they do not dominate. I am confident that he will continue to thrive and, if necessary, learn to manage his allergies independently. If I can facilitate that process in any way and create a healthy environment and attitude within him, I will have done part of my job as his mum.

My hope again is that this book will have helped you and your child on your journey. There are many people to help you and there are many families in similar situations to yours. Whatever stage of the journey you are at, remember that it will change and it will improve. There will be battles ahead but nothing is insurmountable and with some advice and good management your child too will thrive.

Resources

The information in this section is designed to help you in your everyday management of allergy. There are links for baking, shopping and education as well as some useful products that have been referred to throughout the book. There is a vast amount of support accessible through the internet and through charities. I would particularly recommend Allergy UK and the Anaphylaxis Campaign. Both of these are UK-based charities that provide product alerts, a newsletter, a fantastic website, training for families as well as healthcare professionals and support about living with allergies from childhood through to becoming a teenager. Allergy UK's website can be found at www.allergyuk.org and their helpline number is 01322 619898. The Anaphylaxis Campaign website is www.anaphylaxis. org.uk and the helpline number is 01252 542029.

Allergy management

www.cofargroup.org

'Food allergy in children and young people' (2011). National Institute for Health and Care Excellence – http://guidance.nice.org.uk/ CG116

www.bda.uk.com/foodfacts/Allergy.pdf

www.nice.org.uk

'Testing for Food Allergy in Children and Young People' (2011). National Institute for Health and Care Excellence. *Clinical Guidelines* 116, 1–12.

Breastfeeding support

www.breastfeedingnetwork.org.uk
www.laleche.org.uk
www.nhs.uk

Eating out

www.dietarycard.co.uk

Education

www.allergyadventures.com

Books for toddlers

Freddy the Mouse Allergy Education – www.freddythemouse.com
The BugyBops from the Buga Bees series – www.amazon.co.uk

Books for older children

The Itchy Kids Club by Jill Grabowski – www.amazon.co.uk
The *No Biggie Bunch* series – www.amazon.co.uk
One of the Gang by Gina Clowes – www.amazon.co.uk
Note: Medikidz produce a food allergy comic – www.medikidz.com

Food labelling

Allergen avoidance sheet – www.nice.org.uk
www.foodallergens.info
Food Standards Agency – www.food.gov.uk/safereating/allergyintol/label

Food shopping

www.ellaskitchen.co.uk

www.freefromforkids.co.uk
www.goodnessdirect.co.uk
www.organix.com
www.plum-baby.co.uk
www.vegusto.co.uk

Baking

www.bbc.co.uk/food/diets/gluten_free
www.bbc.co.uk/food/diets/nut_free
www.bbc.co.uk/food/diets/dairy_free
www.cakecraftshop.co.uk
www.cozi.com/live-simply/lunch-box-envy-2
www.dennycraftmoulds.co.uk
www.freefromrecipesmatter.com
www.glutendairyfree.co.uk
www.ibakewithout.com
www.lunchboxdoctor.com
www.piginthekitchen.co.uk
www.sweetrosie.wordpress.com
www.theintolerantgourmet.com
www.veganfamily.co.uk

Cakes and puddings

www.lazydayfoods.com
www.mscupcake.co.uk
www.pudology.com

Chocolate and advent calendars

www.kinnerton.com
www.moofreechocolates.com
www.zerozebra.com

Ice cream and smoothies

www.bessantanddrury.com
www.kirstys.co.uk
www.smooze.co.uk
www.swedishglace.com
www.zenzenfood.co.uk

Milk substitutes

www.alpro.co.uk
www.kokodairyfree.com
www.nutricia.co.uk
www.oatly.co.uk

Yoghurts

www.alpro.com/uk
www.coyo.co.uk

Products

www.allerbling.com
www.allerguard.co.uk
www.allermates.com
www.kidsaware.co.uk
www.laurenshope.com
www.mediband.com
www.medicalert.org

Research

www.leapstudy.co.uk

Schools

• •

The Anaphylaxis Campaign website provides a list of possible triggers, top tips on how to conduct a risk assessment and set up a protocol to manage nut allergies in schools, including sample documents in the schools section of their website: www.anaphylaxis.org.uk

The Health Education Trust has developed a best practice guidance tool for 'allergy aware' training in secondary schools. This toolkit can be downloaded from www.healthedtrust.com/pdf/HET-allergy-toolkit.pdf

The trust has produced a policy guide on 'Managing Medicines in Schools', which covers the issues surrounding pupils with food allergies along with asthma, epilepsy and diabetes, and it is available as a free download: www.gov.uk/government/publications/managing-medicines-in-schools-and-early-years-settings/

Support

• •

Get connected through Facebook and blogs. Below are some of the best support groups and websites. Please remember that these sites often reflect the views of their authors and should not take the place of a qualified professional.

www.actionagainstallergy.co.uk
www.allergyuk.org
www.anaphylaxis.org.uk
www.foodallergy.org
www.godairyfree.org
www.kidswithfoodallergies.org
www.mumsnet.com
www.triggerallergy.com

Allergy alerts

Allergy UK – www.allergyuk.org

The American Academy of Allergy Asthma and Immunology – www.aaaai.org

The Anaphylaxis Campaign – www.anaphylaxis.org.uk

Food Standards Agency – www.food.gov.uk

Asthma

www.asthma.org.uk

Autoinjector information and expiry reminders

www.epipen.com

www.jext.co.uk

Eczema

www.eczema.org

Emergency Plans

www.bsaci.org – standard UK emergency plans

> The following two emergency plans are **examples only**. Your child will need an individually tailored plan from a doctor. These ones are only for IgE mediated allergies (see page 4).

Written emergency plan for food allergy suitable for use in pre-school and school – EXAMPLE

Insert child's
photo here

_____[CHILD'S NAME]

is SEVERELY ALLERGIC to
[ALLERGENIC FOODS]

- Please do not let him eat **[ALLERGENIC FOODS]**.
- When baking please do not let him handle **[ALLERGENIC FOODS]**.
- Please do not let him share **[ALLERGENIC FOODS]**.
- He needs **[SAFE FOOD AND DRINK]** at snack time.
- Please wash his hands.

How to spot an allergic reaction:
- Itchy red eyes
- Swelling of lips, face, eyes
- Rash and hives (wheals, blisters or welts) on face or body
- Sickness and/or stomach pain

What to do:
- Stay with [CHILD'S NAME] and call for help.
- Give Piriton (antihistamine). Repeat if vomited.

WATCH FOR SIGNS OF ANAPHYLAXIS

- Difficulty breathing/noisy breathing
- Swelling of tongue
- Swelling of throat
- Difficulty talking/hoarse voice
- Wheeze or persistent cough
- Loss of consciousness/collapse/drowsiness
- Pale or blue and floppy

What to do if there are signs of anaphylaxis:

- Give EpiPen (see below).
- Call 999 – state 'Ambulance required. This is an emergency case of anaphylaxis in a child'.
- If no improvement in five minutes, give second EpiPen.

How to give an EpiPen.

- Form a fist around the EpiPen and pull off grey cap.
- Place black end against outer mid-thigh.
- Push down hard until you hear a click.
- Hold for 10 seconds.
- Remove EpiPen and be careful not to touch needle.
- Massage the needle site for 10 seconds.

- 1st contact: [MOST AVAILABLE PARENT/CARER NAME AND TELEPHONE NUMBER]
- 2nd contact: [OTHER PARENT/CARER NAME AND TELEPHONE NUMBER]

Emergency treatment plan for severe allergic reaction with asthma – EXAMPLE

Date of clinic: ————————————————

TREATMENT PLAN

Insert child's
photo here

Name _____

dob _____

PROBLEM: Allergy to

This child is at risk of a severe allergic reaction.

1. If he eats any of the above by mistake, he should immediately receive Piriton_mg (_× 5 ml teaspoon) [to be completed by child's doctor] followed by 4 puffs of his Ventolin/Bricanyl via a spacer device.

2. If he develops breathing difficulties, noisy breathing, becomes blue, drowsy or unresponsive, he should be given the EpiPen syringe_mg [to be completed by child's doctor] into the outer mid-thigh.

3. If breathing difficulties or EpiPen given, dial 999.

4. If he has not improved within 5–10 minutes, he should be given a second EpiPen and 10 puffs of his Ventolin.

Travel plan – **EXAMPLE**

Personal Details

Date of birth: _____

Full name: _____

Insert child's
photo here

Allergens to be avoided: _____

Prepared by: Dr/Nurse

Signed   Date

Additional information:

This person is at risk of a severe allergic reaction (anaphylaxis) if accidentally exposed to the trigger(s) that cause the allergic reaction.

Emergency medications should be accessible at all times while travelling.

Emergency medications may include one or more of the following: adrenaline autoinjectors (e.g. EpiPen or Jext), antihistamines, immuno-therapy (either Staloral drops or Grazax tablets) and asthma medications, as per their Emergency Plan.

Administration of an adrenaline autoinjector is the first line treatment for anaphylaxis. Adrenaline autoinjectors contain a fixed, single dose of adrenaline and **do not** represent a safety risk.

A safe supply of food and liquids, appropriate for the travel period, should be permitted. The luggage hold of an aircraft is not an appropriate place for emergency medications to be stored as they:

- Need to be immediately available.
- Can be broken with rough handling.
- May be lost if luggage goes astray.
- Should not be subjected to temperature fluctuations.

Diaries

•••

Food Diary for the Dietician

	Milk	Breakfast	Snack	Lunch	Snack	Dinner	Milk
Day 1							
Day 2							
Day 3							
Day 4							
Day 5							
Day 6							
Day 7							
Day 8							
Day 9							
Day 10							
Day 11							
Day 12							
Day 13							
Day 14							

Symptom diary: Immediate Type Allergies

What are the symptoms?	How rapidly did they come and go?	What food was eaten just beforehand? (include major allergens, such as peanuts, tree nuts, milk, egg, wheat, soya, fish, shellfish, sesame, kiwi fruit)	What treatment was given?

Delayed type allergies

Week 0 – Before Milk Exclusion

Symptoms	Day 1	Day 2	Day 3	Day 4	Day 5	Day 6	Day 7
Eczema severity Scale 0–5							
Stools passed							
Stool consistency							
Mucus in stools							
Night-time waking							
Appetite							
Episodes of reflux							
Other							
Other							

During Milk Exclusion – Week 1

Symptoms	Day 1	Day 2	Day 3	Day 4	Day 5	Day 6	Day 7
Eczema severity Scale 0–5							
Stools passed							
Stool consistency							
Mucus in stools							
Night-time waking							
Appetite							
Episodes of reflux							
Other							
Other							

During Milk Exclusion – Week 2

Symptoms	Day 1	Day 2	Day 3	Day 4	Day 5	Day 6	Day 7
Eczema severity Scale 0–5							
Stools passed							
Stool consistency							
Mucus in stools							
Night-time waking							
Appetite							
Episodes of reflux							
Other							
Other							

Milk Fully Reintroduced

Symptoms	Day 1	Day 2	Day 3	Day 4	Day 5	Day 6	Day 7
Eczema severity Scale 0–5							
Stools passed							
Stool consistency							
Mucus in stools							
Night-time waking							
Appetite							
Episodes of reflux							
Other							
Other							

Reading labels

• •

Below is a list of allergens and alternative names to look out for when reading labels. It also details the foods that commonly contain the allergens.*

Food name	Also called	Examples of foods that 'may contain...'
Milk	• Beta-lactoglobulin • Casein, rennet casein • Caseinate (ammonium caseinate, calcium caseinate, magnesium caseinate, potassium caseinate and sodium caseinate) • Delactosed or demineralised whey • Dry milk, milk solids • Hydrolysed casein and hydrolysed milk protein • Lactalbumin and lactalbumin phosphate • Lactose • Lactoferrin, lactoglobulin • Milk derivative, fat and protein • Modified milk ingredients • Whey and whey protein concentrate • Hydrolysed whey • Whey syrup sweetener	• Butter, buttermilk • Cheese, curds • Cream, ice cream • Ghee and butter fat • Kefir (milk drink) • Kumiss (fermented milk drink) • Sour cream • Yoghurt

Food name	Also called	Examples of foods that 'may contain...'
Egg	• Albumin, albumen • Conalbumin • Egg substitutes, for example, Egg Beaters • Globulin • Livetin • Lysozyme • Ovo (means egg), for example, ovalbumin, ovomucin, ovotransferrin • Silico-albuminate • Vitellin • Dried egg • Lecithin (E322) (very rarely, usually soya based) • Ovoglobulin • Ovovitellin	• Baked goods (including some type of breads) and baking mixes • Battered and fried foods • Cream-filled desserts, for example, custards, meringues, puddings and ice creams • Egg and fat substitutes • Fat replacers • Lecithin • Mayonnaise • Meat products with fillers, for example, meatballs and meatloaf • Nougats, marzipan • Pasta (fresh pasta, some types of dry pasta for example, egg noodles) • Quiche, soufflé • Salad dressings, creamy dressings • Sauces, for example, Béarnaise, hollandaise, Newburg, tartar

Food name	Also called	Examples of foods that 'may contain...'
Peanuts	• Arachis oil • Beer nuts • Goober nuts and goober peas • Ground nuts • Kernels • Mandelonas, Nu-Nuts • Nut meats • Valencias • Earth nuts • Manilla nuts • Monkey nuts • Pinda, pinder • Peanut flour/peanut protein	• Ethnic foods, such as satay, Thai, Vietnamese, Chinese, Indian, Middle Eastern, African • Hydrolysed plant protein and vegetable protein • Nut substitutes • Peanut butter • Peanut oil • Vegetarian meat substitutes • Salad dressings • Biscuits, cakes, muesli bars • Breakfast cereals
Fish		• Surimi • Variations of Caesar salad with anchovies • Puttanesca sauce • Gentleman's relish • Worcestershire sauce (contains anchovy) • Caponata • Kedgeree

Food name	Also called	Examples of foods that 'may contain...'
Tree nuts	• Anacardium nuts • Filberts (hazelnuts) • Nut meats • Pinon • Queensland nut (macadamia)	• Dishes such as almond chicken, pad thai and satay • Gianduja and gianduia • Marzipan (almond paste) • Tree nut oils • Pralines • Spreads, for example, almond paste-based spreads, cheese spreads, chocolate nut spreads • Nougat • Nut butter • Nutella • Vegetarian dishes • Processed meat products e.g. coronation chicken • Pesto • Chocolates, biscuits, etc.

Food name	Also called	Examples of foods that 'may contain...'
Soy	• Bean curd, soybean curds • Edamame • Kinako • Natto • Nimame • Okara • Soya, soja, soybean and soyabeans • Soy protein, vegetable protein, soya nuts • Textured soy flour (TSF), textured soy protein (TSP) and textured vegetable protein (TVP) • Yuba • Soya albumin • Lecithin (E322)/soya lecithin • Miso • Soya protein isolate • Tofu • Hydrolysed vegetable protein	• Bean sprouts • Breadcrumbs, cereals and crackers • Breaded foods • Hydrolysed plant protein (HPP), hydrolysed soy protein (HSP) and hydrolysed vegetable protein (HVP) • Imitation dairy food • Child formula, follow-up formula, nutrition supplements for toddlers and children • Meal replacements • Meat products with fillers • Mexican foods, for example, chilli, taco fillings and tamales • Miso • Nutrition supplements • Sauces, for example, soy, shoyu, tamari, teriyaki, Worcestershire • Simulated fish and meat products • Stews • Tempeh • Vegetarian dishes

Food name	Also called	Examples of foods that 'may contain...'
Wheat	• Durum wheat, spelt, Kamut • Couscous • Bran, wheat bran, wheatgerm, wheat gluten • Farina • Rusk • Semolina, durum wheat semolina • Flour, wholewheat flour, wheat flour, wheat starch • Starch, modified starch, hydrolysed starch, food starch, edible starch • Vegetable starch, vegetable gum, vegetable protein • Cereal filler, cereal binder, cereal protein • All cereals of *Triticum* genus • *Triticum spelta* L. (spelt) • *Triticum poloniwum* L.C (Polish wheat) • *Triticum turgidum* (Kamut)	• Bread and baked foods: many rye and corn loaves contain some wheat. Pitta, crumpets, muffins, tortillas, tacos, doughnuts, cakes, cookies, biscuits, crackers, croutons, packet snacks, rusks, waffles, pancakes, crepes, pizzas, pretzels, breadsticks, communion wafers, pasta and pastry. Also Yorkshire pudding, suet pudding and many other puddings • Cereals: most cereals will contain some wheat. The exceptions are porridge oats, corn flakes, rice krispies and granola. Always read the labels • Flour and pasta: all of these will contain some wheat unless stated to be wheat free or buckwheat, which is not from the wheat family • Meat and fish: burgers, rissoles, salami, sausages, corned beef, luncheon meat, liver-sausage, continental sausages, pâtés, meat and fish pastes and spreads, ham, fish and Scotch eggs and other breaded meats and poultry

Food name	Also called	Examples of foods that 'may contain...'
Wheat continued		• Vegetable products: vegetable pâtés and spreads, vegetables coated in breadcrumbs, vegetables tempura, tinned beans, soups and tinned and packet snack or ready-prepared foods
		• Sauces and condiments: gravy, packet, jar and bottled sauces, casserole and ready-meal mixes, stock cubes and granules, ready-prepared mustard, stuffing, baking powder, monosodium glutamate, some spice mixes
		• Desserts: most puddings, pastry, yoghurts containing cereal, ice cream, pancakes, cheesecakes and others with a biscuit base
		• Beverages: malted milk, chocolate, Ovaltine and other powdered drinks
		• Sweets: liquorice, chocolate, chocolate bars and most wrapped bars. Other sweets (check labels)
		• Medication: many prescribed and over-the-counter drugs contain wheat
		• Other: glue on labels and postage stamps

Food name	Also called	Examples of foods that 'may contain...'
Sesame	• Benne, benne seed and benniseed • Gingelly and gingelly oil • Seeds • Sesamol and sesamolina • *Sesamum indicum* • Simsim • Til	• Bread, breadcrumbs and sticks, cereals, crackers, melba toast and muesli • Dips and spreads • Ethnic foods, for example, flavoured rice, noodles, shish kebabs, stews and stir fries • Sesame oil, sesame salt (gomasio) • Tahini (sesame paste) • Tempeh • Vegetarian burgers

Food name	Also called	Examples of foods that 'may contain...'
Shellfish	• Clams • Mussels • Scallops • Oysters • Winkles • Some crustaceans commonly eaten are shrimp, prawn, lobster, crayfish and crabs	• Ceviche • Cioppino • Callaloo • Clam chowder • Curanto • Fruits de mer • Paella • Sashimi • Shrimp cocktail • Lobster bisque • She-crab soup • Sliced fish soup • Sushi Check the following: • Caponata (Sicilian relish) • Gelatin if derived from fish bones • Marshmallows depending on gelatin used • Pizza toppings • Salad dressings • Sauces • Spreads • Deli meats • Hot dogs (from gelatin) • Compost or fertilisers • Lip balm and gloss • Pet food

*Lists adapted from www.kidswithfoodallergies.org

References

American Academy of Pediatrics – www.aap.org

British Dietetic Association Paediatric Group, 2010 – www.bda.uk.com
Clark, A. T., Skypala, I., Leech, S. C., Ewan, P. W., Dugu'e, P., Brathwaite, N., Huber, P. A. J. and Nasser, S. M. (2010). 'British Society for Allergy and Clinical Immunology guidelines for the management of egg allergy'. *Clinical & Experimental Allergy*, 40 (8).

'Community-based Strategies for Breastfeeding Promotion and Support in Developing Countries'. World Health Organization. 2003.

Fitzsimons, R., Gibbs, L. and Fox, A. T. (2010). 'Food Allergy in Children'. *Practice Nurse*, 39 (10), 39–45.

Fitzsimons, R., Kane, P. and Fox, A. T. (2009). 'Anaphylaxis part 3: Managing Emergenicies with Confidence'. *British Journal of School Nursing*, 4 (8), 218–224.

Fitzsimons, R., Kane, P. and Fox, A. T. (2012). 'Anaphylaxis: Managing Emergencies in School'. *British Journal of Nursing*, 7 (3), 65–69.

'Food Allergy and Intolerance Specialist Group. Cow's Milk Free Diet for Infants and Children'. British Dietetic Association, 2012.

'Guidelines for the Diagnosis and Management of Food Allergy', published in 2010 *Journal of Allergy and Clinical Immunology*, 126 (6); supplement S1–56.

Holloway, E., Fox, A. T. and Fitzsimons, R. (2011). 'Diagnosing and Managing Food Allergy in Children'. *Practitioner*, 255 (1741), 19–22.

Leung, James, S. C. and Leung, Alexander, K. C. (2010), *Food Allergy*.

Leung, D. Y., Sampson, H. A., Yunginger, J. W., Burks, A. W. Jr, Schneider, L. C., Wortel, C. H., Davis, F. M., Hyun, J. D., Shanahan, W. R. Jr (2003). 'Effect of Anti-IgE therapy in patients with peanut allergy'. *New England Journal of Medicine* 348 (11): 986–993.

Pumphrey, R. (2004). Anaphylaxis: 'Can we tell who is at risk of a Fatal Reaction?' *Current Opinion in Allergy and Clinical Immunology* 4: 285–290.

Sicherer, S. H. *Understanding and Managing Your Child's Food Allergies*. (2006). A John Hopkins Press Health Book.

Staden, U., Rolinck-Werninghaus ,C., Brewe, F., Wahn, U., Niggermann, B., Beyer, K. (2007). 'Specific oral tolerance induction in food allergy in children: efficacy and clinical patterns to reaction'. *Allergy* 62 (11): 1261–1269.

Swan, K. E., Fitzsimons, R., Boardman, A. and Fox, A. T. (2012). 'The Prevention and Management of Anaphylaxis'. *Paediatrics and Child Health*.

Tariq, S. M., Matthews, S. M., Hakim, E. A. and Arshad, S. H. (2000). 'Egg Allergy in Infancy predicts Respiratory Allergic Disease by 4 Years of Age'. *Pediatric Allergy Immunology* 11 (3), 162–167.

'Testing for Food Allergy in Children and Young People (2011)'. National Institute for Health and Care Excellence. Clinical Guideline 116, 1–12. www.nice.org.uk

'Britain's Top 100 Children's Doctors'. *The Times Magazine*. Times Newspapers Limited 2013.

'Britain's Top 250 Consultants by Specialty'. *Tatler Doctors Guide 2013*. Conde Nast UK 2013.

'Vaccines against Allergies'. *Current Topics in Microbiology and Immunology* (352) edited by Valenta, R. and Coffman, R. L. Springer (2011).

Index